WONDER HERBS

A Guide to Three Adaptogens

J.P. Saleeby, MD

To order additional copies of this book, contact:
Xlibris Corporation
1-888-795-4274
www.Xlibris.com
Orders@Xlibris.com
32822

Contents

Active Ingredients

Usual Doses

Side Effects and Toxicity

Brief History of Jiaogulan

How Jiaogulan is used
Regulation of Blood Pressure
Regulation of Blood Lipids
Improving Circulation and Cardiovascular function
Boosting the Immune System
Support of Liver Function
Lowering Blood Glucose
Enhancing Athletic Performance
Avoiding the Signs of Aging
Reducing Risk of Cancer
Other Benefits of Jiaogulan

Active Ingredients

Usual Doses

Side Effects and Toxicity

Drug / Herbal Interaction

*This book is dedicated to my children
Michael and Madison*

Notice

This book is intended as a reference volume and not a medical manual. The information given here is designed to help the reader make informed decisions about the use of Adaptogen herbs. All dosages and usage of the herbs mentioned in this book are what the typical experienced herbalist is likely to prescribe.

The statements regarding herbs have not been evaluated by the Food and Drug Administration. These statements are not intended to diagnose, treat, cure or prevent any disease.[†]

Mention of specific companies, organizations or authorities in this book does not imply endorsement by the author. Dr. Saleeby receives no monetary compensation for mention of any products (excluding VSN and SSN products) in this book.

Internet addresses and web references in this book were accurate at the time this book went to press.

[†]   This statement is in compliance with FDA regulations.

Special Thanks to Amber Keefer, Angela Kaylor,
RN MPH & Sharon Coopersmith, RRT
for their writing, reviewing, editing, and critique.

Introduction

JP Saleeby, MD

In humanities never ending search for the magic cure-all, many a snake oil salesman in modern times has become wealthy. Attempting to separate the chaff from the grain, searching for the panacea of health, the consumer is bogged down in a quagmire of products most of which do not work. Take for instance supplement infomercials that run for a couple of months then all of a sudden disappear after accomplishing the goal of stuffing the bank accounts of their promoters. The supplement industry is a billion-dollar a year business. To this day after starting my nutritional medicine practice in 1998, I have been deluged with email and junk mail from companies wanting me to "sell" their products by whatever scheme (usually multi-level-marketing) to the consumer (my patient).

The Dietary Supplement Health and Education Act of 1994 often referred to as DSHEA took the FDA out of the business of policing the dietary supplement industry. This law has its ups and downs. On the downside for consumers there is no governing body to regulate what a product promoter can claim about a particular supplement. So caveat emptor, let the buyer beware. The Internet offers the lay public the opportunity to research the subject, but alas the Internet is infested with misinformation. The upside to DSHEA is lower prices for consumers. No need for tremendous expenditures for Research & Development in "proving for the FDA" the efficacy and safety of supplements, thus the cost to consumers is very low compared with many pharmaceuticals. Also this serves the supplement industry with great profits. That is what prompted me to research and formulate a supplement line for use with my patients following many of my protocols for wellness. The result was a safe pharmaceutical-grade bioavailable nutracutical at low cost to the consumer. Something I could recommend and sleep well at night knowing I had done good for my patients.

It must be human nature to be easily swayed by fancy advertisers and convincing charismatic spokesmen that deliver a message of the miracle potion to ensure health, wellness or weight loss. So I do my part as a physician to inform my patients what is correct and backed by scientific research, not by whimsical belief. Time and time again I am assaulted by late night infomercials that boast the latest trend or "hot" supplement to bestow good health. It is this reckless and un-policed forum that has prompted me to put some of my thoughts to paper for those who don't have the luxury of sitting across from me in consultation. This remains the reason I maintain an online blog and have written this book.

As I spent the last few years researching and writing for this book, I considered writing the world-renowned herbalist and integrative practitioner Dr. Andrew Weil for a forward to this book. I later decided against this move, as there is really no need for any forward and certainly not a need for an Imprimatur. No need for any sanctioning individual, body or colleges to lend credence to what I have done. What gives me license to write on this topic? Well there is no residency training or credentialing process that affords legitimacy here in this country, so the reader must take into account my many years of self-study and personal research in the field as well as my fifteen years of practicing clinical medicine. I a certain this is enough to produce credible text. Enough to offer the reader comfort in what is expressed within these pages is evidenced-based fact rather than fiction. This represents the work of a scientist unlike the un-credentialed talking heads on those late-night infomercials. This remains an easy to read, moderately technical (but not overwhelmingly so) book so the casual lay reader may enjoy it as much as the medical upper or mid-level practitioner who is attempting to gain an entry level understanding of these remarkable herbs for their practice of medicine.

As a medical practitioner my allopathic training in traditional western medicine taught that healing or curing came about by identifying the root cause of a disease and eliminating it. This is more commonly known as the "doctrine of a specific etiology of disease". In the East another approach was developed thousands of year ahead and is centered on the disruption of the balance within and the assistance with herbals or other remedies to restore balance. This practice allows the body to cure itself.

For over a decade and a half I have witnessed first hand the ravishes of disease, obesity, lack of exercise, and poor nutrition. I have seen what the effects of a stressful lifestyle can have on the body. I have treated many successfully. Those that are disciplined and listen and follow appropriately mapped out programs reap the best results. Those that grow tired of the rituals of good health fall to the wayside and eventually live a lesser quality of life, or even succumb to a premature death.

Obviously there is no substitute for proper nutrition & hydration, adequate sleep, aerobic and resistance exercise and a balanced neuro-endocrine system. I am not going to elaborate on this subject as much research has proven its effectiveness. Many books and articles belabor the benefits.

Rather I am going to focus on a more esoteric subject, that of a select subset of medicinal herbs that will embellish and enhance an already well oiled machine. Once a person has committed to proper diet, exercise and rest; once a person has committed to selected dietary supplements it is time for the next step. As you cannot put the cart before the horse here, I do not advise continued cigarette smoking with the use of herbs as a quick-fix to lowering lung cancer risk. Smoke cessation first, then consider this as the next step.

There is a class of herbs that aid our bodies in adapting to environmental changes. Whether the environmental changes are emotional stress, physical stress, toxins, or a drastic change in our exercise program or work schedule, these herbs exert a balancing effect. They are known collectively as adaptogens or adaptogen herbs. Only about one in every 300 herbs is considered an adaptogen. The most commonly recognized adaptogen herb has to be Panax ginseng. This is the benchmark herb that all other adaptogens are compared.

The term adaptogen was coined in 1947 by a Russian toxicologist and pharmacologist named Dr. Nikolai Vasilyevich Lazarev. As the father of modern day research into adaptogen herbs, Dr. Lazarev set up some basic criteria that must be met in order for consideration in this very special class of herbs:

1. It must cause only minimal disruption in the body's physiological functions;
2. It must increase the body's resistance to adverse influences not by a specific action but by a wide range of physical, chemical, and biochemical factors;
3. It must have an overall normalizing effect, improving all kinds of conditions and aggravating none. And it must restore balance to the system regardless of the

direction of the illness (for example, an adaptogen would work equally well in a depleted condition as it would in a condition of excess).

Herbalists believe adaptogens work by supporting adrenal function enabling cells access to more energy and helping them eliminate toxic metabolic byproducts. Adaptogens also help the body use oxygen more efficiently and improve the regulation of the body's natural rhythms. Though they all work in these similar ways, each adaptogen has a distinct personality and unique medicinal qualities. We will visit what I consider three rather remarkable yet generally lesser known of adaptogen herbs. They are, in no evident order: Rhodiola rosea, Eleuthero (Eleutherococcus senticosus) and Jiaogulan (Gynostemma pentaphyllum).

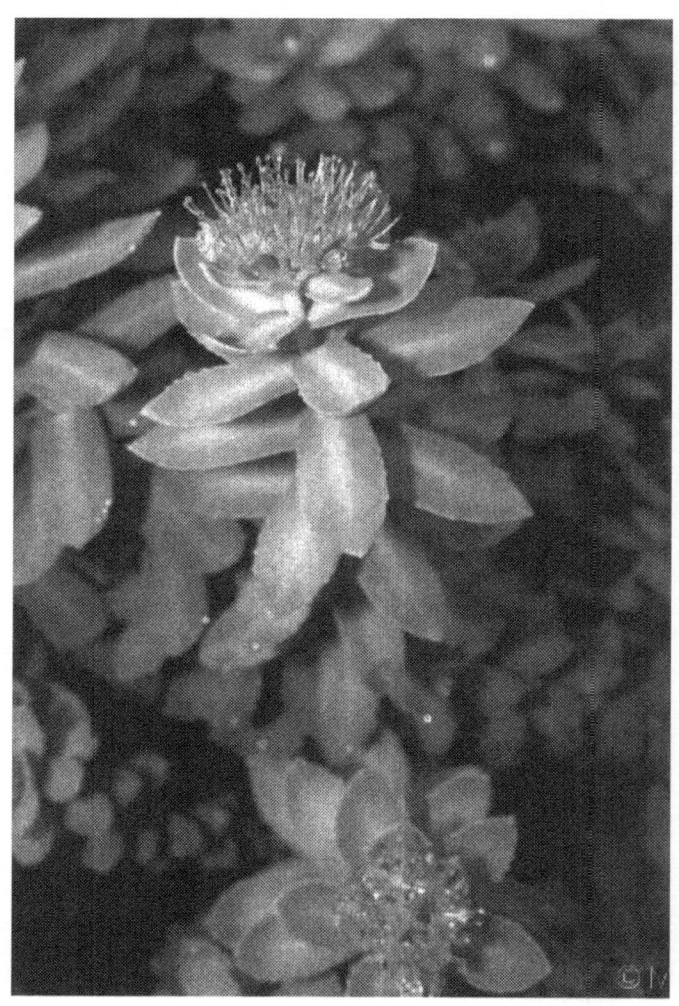

Rhodiola rosea

Chapter I

Rhodiola Rosea

JP Saleeby, MD and Amber Keefer

What Are Adaptogens and How Do They Work?

A unique class of herbal products called adaptogens has the broadest range of healing properties of any herbal medicine, but their unique value is that they specifically relieve or reduce the effects of stress on our body systems. In 1947, a Russian scientist named Dr. Nikolai V. Lazarev, first coined the word adaptogen. As can be inferred from the word itself, an adaptogen is a natural plant substance that helps the body to adapt or cope with all types of stresses including trauma and injury, sleeplessness, depression, psychological stress, environmental stress, and infection.

For centuries, people around the world have been using herbal remedies to help their bodies deal with the effects of stress. Ancient cultures revered adaptogenic herbs like Rhodiola rosea for their stress-enhancing properties. Adaptogens work by building up an energy reserve to be tapped into when the body needs it most, helping to correct whatever is out of balance. By doing so, they enhance an individual's ability to cope with different kinds of stress.

Although Dr. Lazarev was one of the first to report on several indigenous plants that help increase the body's natural resistance to environmental stresses, several clinical trials have provided strong evidence that Rhodiola rosea extract possesses positive mood enhancing and anti-stress properties with no detectable levels of toxicity. Soviet researchers classified Rhodiola rosea as a 'second generation adaptogen' (due to its chronological discovery) because of its ability to increase resistance to a variety of chemical, biological and physical stresses. The benefits of Rhodiola rosea are believed to include antidepressant, anticancer, cardio-protective and central nervous system enhancement. I have used the term "believed" here because of the paucity of published scientific study reasonably "proving" the effects or outcomes. Regardless, those few studies seem to indicate that the herb may be useful in treating sleep difficulties, poor appetite, irritability, hypertension, headaches and fatigue following intense physical or intellectual strain.

Western science is now taking a closer look at how adaptogens can increase the body's ability to cope with internal and external stress factors. Adaptogens help maintain the stable internal environment inside the body known as homeostasis. One of their most important characteristics, however, is that they are safe, possessing few known side effects. An adaptogen is non-toxic and non-habit forming, possessing a wide range of therapeutic benefits that must benefit the body without doing it harm. The main effects of adaptogens are an increased availability of energy during the day, decreased stress, increased endurance, greater mental alertness and deep, restful sleep. Adaptogens have also been known to significantly accelerate the recovery process after illness.

Unlike allopathic drugs that carry with them the possibility of side effects, adaptogens are natural nutrients and are found in a rather few types of plants. For the purpose of this book we will discuss Rhodiola rosea, Eleutherococcus senticosus and Gynostemma pentaphyllum. Additionally I will remark on some comparisons to the landmark adaptogen herb recognized by most Americans as ginseng (Panax ginseng).

Adaptogenic herbals are believed to nourish the internal organs by increasing the blood supply through increased cardiac output. They are also believed to normalize the nervous and hormonal systems in the body when they are adversely affected by stress. The body's way of helping itself cope in times of stress is to produce the hormones epinephrine (also called adrenaline), which triggers a flight or fight response and norepinephrine (also called noradrenaline), which is important in maintaining wakefulness and alertness. When norepinephrine levels are low, depression can set in along with fatigue. Both hormones are produced in the adrenal medulla. (Refer to Table 2 in Appendix)

By enhancing the functions of the sympathetic and parasympathetic systems, Rhodiola rosea enables the body to put out more energy during stress while at the same time maintaining higher energy reserves.

Dopamine, a precursor to adrenaline and norepinephrine plays an important role in normal body movements. Consuming sugar, tea, coffee, chocolate, alcohol or smoking a cigarette can also trigger the release of dopamine, which converts to higher levels of epinephrine and norepinephrine. Other safer alternatives to the aforementioned are natural adaptogens, eating a well-balanced diet, regular exercise and getting plenty of rest.

It is important to note, however, that adaptogens can influence each individual differently. They are not normal stimulants, but if you are mentally exhausted or physically fatigued, adaptogens may help you feel more energetic and revitalized. Although they are not tranquilizers, they can help you relax and make life easier to cope with without having a drug-like hangover effect on the body. Not many plants possess adaptogenic properties. In fact, it is estimated that only one in 4,000 plants (1 in 300 herbs) are classified as an adaptogen.

Adaptogen Deficiency

Adaptogens not only help us cope with stress and the hassles of every day living; they are also powerful antioxidants. The antioxidants contained in adaptogens help the body fight free radicals that are released during the oxidative process of metabolism in the body. This process results in a variety of problems such as cell degeneration, cancer, aging and many chronic diseases.

It is reported in the scientific literature that endurance can be increased by up to 26% and an increase in strength by nearly 10% with the adaptogen Rhodiola. Many bodybuilders and athletes supplement with adaptogens to improve their performance and help the body return quicker to its normal resting state making it a viable alternative to other more harmful ergogenic aids.

Safety of Adaptogens

Adaptogens are completely safe (by definition) when taken within the prescribed dose range, effective and contain no drugs, preservatives or banned substances. That being said, Rhodiola rosea (a second-generation adaptogen) has been found to be four times less potentially toxic than Korean ginseng (a first generation adaptogen) at extremely high doses. First and second generation adaptogens are categorized as such based on their discovery and/or use as adaptogens chronologically.

Brief History of Rhodiola rosea

Rhodiola rosea, more commonly known as Golden Root, nd also known as Arctic Root, belongs to the plant family Crassulaceae. Rhodiola rosea grows primarily in dry, sandy soil at high altitudes in the arctic areas of Europe and Asia, (particularly Eastern Siberia), where the plant has been used medicinally for centuries.

The Rhodiola rosea plant reaches a height of about 12 to 30 inches and produces yellow blossoms. It is a perennial herbaceous with red, pink or yellowish flowers and a thick rhizome (bulb) that is fragrant when cut. Although the herb has no biological relation to the common rose, it has a similar fragrance, hence the name.

Using Rhodiola rosea for curative purposes dates as far back as the early centuries. The Greek physician, Dioscorides, first recorded medicinal applications of rodia riza in 77AD. It was not until 1961, when G.V. Krylov, a renowned Russian botanist, identified the Golden Root (or Roseroot as it was sometimes called referring to the rose-like fragrance of the fresh cut rootstock) as Rhodiola rosea.

Rhodiola rosea has long been used in the traditional medicine of European and Asian countries for the treatment of depression and anxiety. The Soviet government had conventionally given Rhodiola rosea to its cosmonauts, military and professional athletes as an effective ergogenic aid to help improve their cognitive functions and increase physical performance. Although little is known about this herb in the United States today, because of its remarkable mood enhancing and antidepressant properties, R. rosea is becoming increasingly popular in the West.

Beneficial effects of Rhodiola rosea as shown in studies:

- *Helping to maintain energy levels and increasing stamina*
- *Improving endurance levels*
- *Activating lipase in long distance runners and swimmers*
- *Assisting in the body's protein metabolism*
- *Increasing attention span*
- *Enhancing memory & mental performance*
- *Increasing physical strength & mobility Increasing oxygen circulation to the brain and muscles*
- *Protecting against heart attacks*
- *Shortening the length of recovery time after high intensity workouts*
- *Helping to fight depression by naturally enhancing mood*
- *Lowering stress levels and increasing feelings of well-being*
- *Aiding in the loss of body fat*
- *Removing ammonia from the body*
- *Optimizing serotonin, dopamine and other neuro-transmitter levels in the brain*

In traditional folk medicine, Rhodiola rosea was used to increase physical endurance, work productivity and longevity. Research into Rhodiolia's use conducted by renowned herbologist Dr. I. I. Brekhman (1969) and later by Dr. C. Germano et. al. (1999) found this herb was used to treat depression, fatigue, anemia, impotence, gastrointestinal ailments, infections and nervous system disorders.

For centuries, Chinese emperors sent expeditions to Siberia to bring back these rare natural plants for medicinal preparations. In Middle Asia, Rhodiola rosea tea was the most effective treatment for cold and flu during the severe Asian winters. Mongolian doctors commonly prescribed it for tuberculosis and cancer. Vikings believed the herb enhanced their physical strength and endurance. Carl Linnaeus (1707-1778), often referred to as the father of taxonomy wrote about Rhodiola rosea being used as an astringent and for the treatment of hernia, impotence, hysteria and headache. Even today, Siberians claim that drinking Rhodiola rosea tea will help you to live to be more than 100 years of age.

Still little was known about Rhodiola rosea until the 1930's when it was studied more intently. Between 1725 and 1960, various medicinal applications of Rhodiola rosea appeared in the scientific literature of Sweden, Norway, France, Germany, the Soviet Union and Iceland. In 1947, Russian scientists determined that the herb actually helped increase the body's resistance to numerous environmental stressors. German researchers described the benefits of Rhodiola rosea for pain, headache, scurvy and hemorrhoids. It was also prescribed as a stimulant and anti-inflammatory. The flood of information coming westward about Rhodiola rosea in recent decades after the fall of the Soviet Union is what has sparked increased interest in the plant today.

The Role of Rhodiola rosea in ATP and Creatine Production

Since 1960, more than 180 pharmacological, phytochemical and clinical studies have been published, primarily in European and Slavic languages. In the 1960's, in an effort to train elite athletes for international sports competition, the Soviet Unionspent millions of dollars on research devoted solely to identifying naturally occurring substances that would help increase strength and endurance.

Over the years, Soviet scientists have contributed a wealth of research and knowledge to modern athletic performance. Much of this research was devoted to natural herbs and substances that are found only in Russia and central Asia. In many Russian studies, Rhodiola rosea was shown to increase both strength and muscle mass by affecting the amount of oxygen available for prolonged physical exertion. The herb has also demonstrated the ability to speed recovery time, not only from strenuous training, but also from muscle strains and more serious sports injuries. Rhodiola rosea may well be a safe, natural alternative for body builders, weight lifters and other athletes to anabolic steroids.

According to researcher Dr. A. I. Baranov in an article in the Journal of Ethnopharmacology (1982), information released from the Moscow Institute of Physical Culture (Russia's leading center of athletic performance research) boasts Rhodiola's effect on ATP production. Rhodiola rosea extract has been shown to significantly increase muscle adenosine triphosphate (ATP) and creatine phosphate (CP) levels by increasing the levels of energy-rich fatty acids released from adipose tissue.

Creatine is an important amino acid, a combination of the three amino acids arginine, glycine, and methionine. Like the building blocks that make up proteins, the body either produces it naturally, or it is obtained directly from the foods we eat. On average, the body goes through about 2 grams of creatine each day. Creatine increases the energy content of muscle cells by increasing the availability of ATP (adenosine tri-phosphate), the cells' energy molecule. The amount of strength we have depends on how quickly ATP can be made available during exercise. Most of our body's creatine is contained within skeletal muscle, although some is also present in the heart, brain and testes. When ingested and following the digestive process, creatine is transported into our muscles where it provides additional energy.

Other sources of energy like carbohydrates and fat take longer to convert into energy we can use. But during intense exercise when the body needs a quick source of energy, more ATP in your system means more fuel for your muscles.

Since the human body uses these high-energy phosphate compounds as major sources of energy, increasing the amount of oxygen circulated to the brain and muscles boosts a person's energy level. Unfortunately, the supply of creatine in the body's muscles is not limitless. The average human has between 3.5 and 4 grams of creatine per kilogram of muscle. Once you use up the creatine in a muscle, you then have to rest the muscle and recover before you can exercise it again. However, studies suggest that Rhodiola rosea may increase ATP production in all cells.

Extracts of the Rhodiola rosea root have been found to contain powerful adaptogens. The quest for new medicines to treat diseases like cancer and radiation sickness, as well as to enhance physical and mental performance led to the discovery of a group of phenylpropanoids that are specific to the Rhodiola rosea plant. Despite the various health-promoting effects of Rhodiola rosea being broadly studied abroad, the medicinal benefits of this herb remain largely unknown in the West until recently.

Combating Stress and Fatigue

Rhodiola rosea may be helpful in increasing energy and decreasing mental fatigue. According to the American Academy of Family Physicians and the Russian Department of Family Care, about two-thirds of all office visits are related to stress. Many healthcare professionals now believe that the effects of excessive stress in modern life may lead to chronic states of fatigue-related depression. This is an unfortunate fact, yet reports estimate that about 80% of all illness can be traced back to stress and depression. The power of Rhodiola rosea to help the body adapt to stress may lie in its ability to enhance the level of serotonin, dopamine and other brain neurotransmitters. It's proven effectiveness for depression led Soviet clinicians to use it in combination with antidepressants. Studies showed that a patient's general activity, intellectual and physical productivity levels increased while length of stay in the hospital and side effects associated with tricyclic antidepressants (TCA) decreased.

One study by Dr. A. A. Spasov et. al. (2000) investigated the stimulating and normalizing effect of Rhodiola rosea extract SHR-5 in students during a stressful examination period. The students took the test herbal extract and the placebo for 20 days during an examination period. Both their physical and mental performances were assessed before and after the period, based on objective as well as on subjective evaluation. The most significant improvement in the group taking the Rhodiola rosea extract was seen in physical fitness, mental fatigue and neuro-motor abilities. The self-assessment of the general well being was also significantly better in this group. Another study by Dr. V Darbinyan et. al. (2000) using a group of 56 young, healthy doctors working the night shift in a hospital investigated the effect of repeated low-dose treatment with a standardized extract of rhizome Rhodiola rosea on fatigue during night duty. The effect was measured as total mental performance calculated on a standardized fatigue index for more objective analysis. The tests chosen reflected an overall level of mental fatigue, involving complex perceptive and cognitive cerebral functions such as associative thinking, short-term memory, calculation and ability of concentration and speed of audio-visual perception. A statistically significant improvement in these tests was observed in the treatment group during the first two weeks. No side effects were reported. The results under this well designed study prove scientifically that the rhizome Rhodiola rosea reduces general fatigue under certain stressful conditions.

Effects on the Central Nervous System

The systematic study of the pharmacological effects of Rhodiola rosea, begun in 1965, found that small and medium doses had a simulating effect on lab mice. In contrast, larger doses were found to have more sedative effects while small doses appeared to increase the bioelectrical activity of the brain. Further studies showed that medium range doses, unlike tranquilizers, enhanced the development of conditioned avoidance reflexes in rats and facilitated learning based on emotionally positive reinforcement. Overall, in small and medium doses, Rhodiola rosea stimulated norepinephrine, dopamine, serotonin and nicotinic cholinergic effects in the central nervous system. It also enhanced the effects of these neurotransmitters on the brain by increasing the permeability of the blood brain barrier to precursors of dopamine and serotonin.

Since the neurotransmitter acetylcholine contributes to memory function, agents that block acetylcholine suppress the activity of these ascending pathways and interfere with memory. Rhodiola rosea reverses this blockade. The deterioration of these systems with age results in age-associated memory loss. Therefore, Rhodiola rosea may prevent or ameliorate some age-related dysfunction in these neuronal systems.

Effects on the Immune System

Rhodiola rosea is believed to aid the immune system in two ways. First, it directly stimulates one of the most important kinds of immune cells—Natural Killer (NK) cells that seek and destroy infected cells in the body. Rhodiola rosea works to stabilize the immune system by improving T-cell immunity, thereby, increasing the body's resistance to toxins that may accumulate when an infection develops.

Rhodiola rosea also strengthens the immune system by making a person less susceptible to stress. Scientists have found that stress suppresses immunity and destroys our resistance to various forms of bacterial, fungal or virus attacks. Research indicates Rhodiola rosea may prevent the suppression of B-cell immunity that can occur during stress. It helps to understand that when we are under stress, much of our body's energy is expended. When we are chronically exposed to stress, our other body systems are continuously being robbed of energy. As a result, the body's immunity and resistance to infection are lowered, and we experience fatigue.

Effects on Cardiovascular Health

In a Russian study in 1994 by Dr. L.V. Maslova, et. al., an extract of Rhodiola rosea was found to prevent stress induced cardiac damage. Simultaneously, the extract was determined to prevent both stress-induced release of proteins and higher enzyme levels, which can ultimately damage heart tissue. The findings suggest anti-stressor and cardio protective benefits of Rhodiola rosea without harmful effects on other systems.

Could Rhodiola rosea prevent heart attacks and how? Stress causes adrenaline release that over time produce untoward effects by a complex mechanism referred to as the "adrenal burn" of the heart. Overly contracted heart muscle fibers show contraction bands, a sign of heart muscle damage found in 86% of heart attack victims. Rhodiola rosea appears to decrease the amount of adrenaline and cortisol released during stress, protecting the heart against this adrenaline burn.

Published studies [L.A. Maimeskulova (1998) & I.B. Lishmanov (1993/1997)] have shown that Rhodiola rosea normalizes the heart rate immediately after intense exercise and may also help to decrease blood pressure and lessen irregular heartbeats. It protects against arrhythmias (abnormal heartbeats) by increasing endorphins, our natural opiates that regulate heart rate. The herb also lowers serum fats and cholesterol to some degree while increasing the resistance of blood vessels to cholesterol plaques—yet another significant cardiac "plus" that Rhodiola rosea offers.

Rhodiola rosea to Fight Cancer

Rhodiola rosea shows some promise for combating cancer. Anti-tumor and anti-metastatic effects of Rhodiola rosea extract were established in experiments on laboratory mice and rats with transplantable NK/Ly tumor, Ehrlich's adenocarcinoma, melanoma B16 and Lewis lung carcinoma. Application of a preparation containing Rhodiola rosea was followed by an increase in survival of laboratory animals.

In one human study [O. A. Bocharova, et. al. (1995)], oral administration of Rhodiola rosea extract to 12 patents with superficial bladder carcinoma (T1G1-2) improved the characteristics of the urothelial tissue integration, parameters of leukocyte integrins and T-cell immunity. There needs to be more funding into the study of oncology to find out how far-reaching this herb will be in the fight against cancers. We can only make educated speculations at this point.

Rhodiola rosea and Weight Loss

Clinicians already know that adequate amounts of serotonin help to lift your mood and overall feeling of well-being, as well as decrease your carbohydrate cravings. Rhodiola rosea appears to stimulate fat burning without any side effects. It helps your body increase serotonin production while boosting metabolic rate, a two pronged attack in a war against obesity. The herb also increases hemoglobin and red blood cell levels while favorable changing the muscle to fat ratio of the body.

In a placebo-controlled study [Ramazanov, Zakir, et. al. (1999)], 121 subjects were given either Rhodiola rosea extract or a placebo. The serum lipid levels of those participating in the study were tested at rest and after one hour of exercise. The Rhodiola group had 6% greater serum fatty acid levels than the placebo group at rest, and 44% greater levels after one hour of exercise. This difference is presumably due to the herb's ability to activate adipose lipase, a key enzyme required to burn the body's fat stores.

Similarly, a clinical study at the Georgian State Hospital (in the former Soviet Union) treated 130 overweight patients for 90 days. Afterward, it was found that among those who were given the Rhodiola rosea extract, 92% lost an average of 20 pounds, while the placebo group lost only 8 pounds on the same diet. Recent research has also reported that overweight people have lowered immunity. Researchers attribute this to deficiencies in antioxidants and various nutrients. No matter what weight loss program or system suits your fancy, Rhodiola rosea should be used to augment effective weight (fat) loss. It will also protect your pituitary-adrenal axis system during the process [Hiai, S, et. al.(1979), Fulder, S, et. Al (1981)].

Rhodiola rosea as an Antioxidant

Rhodiola rosea is rich in phenolic compounds, known to have strong antioxidant properties. As an antioxidant, it should help protect the nervous system from oxidative damage by free radicals. Stress interferes with memory functions, and over time, causes deterioration in memory systems. Rhodiola rosea is believed to enhance cognitive functions, learning and memory by stimulating norepinephrine, dopamine, serotonin and acetylcholine neuronal systems. The dual action of cognitive stimulation and emotional calming creates benefits for both immediate cognitive and memory performance and for the long-term preservation of brain functions.

Rhodiola therapy could in fact protect hypoxia-induced biological changes by increasing intracellular oxygen diffusion and efficiency of oxygen utilization. Alternatively, it reduces hypoxia-induced oxidative damage by its antioxidant activities.

Other Benefits of Rhodiola rosea

In diabetics, Rhodiola rosea stimulates the production of more insulin and protects the liver against toxins. Clinical studies indicate that the herb may help prevent the development of hyperglycemia. This is important news for diabetics. In animal experiments, Rhodiola rosea increased blood insulin and decreased glucagon. Test results have shown a 50 to 80% increase in liver glycogen where excess sugar is stored.

Taking Rhodiola rosea as a supplement may also help build greater immunity against bacterial and viral attack, including deadly infections like Anthrax and Smallpox. Annual influenza virus concerns can be thwarted, because the best defense against viruses is having a robust immune system. Rhodiola rosea represents itself as a good adjuvant therapy to yearly immunizations.

In addition, there have been studies indicating that Rhodiola rosea can help patients with sexual dysfunction [Sinclair S, (2000)] and menopausal-related disorders. More research into this is needed before recommendations can comfortably be prescribed.

Who should consider using Rhodiola?

- Anyone who is subject to the depression and/or anxiety
- Anyone seeking increased mental alertness
- Those prone to Alzheimer's or other neurological disease
- Athletes
- Those suffering from degenerative illness or those ravaged by old age

Rhodiola rosea versus Ginseng

Rhodiola rosea has all the advantages of ginseng and eleutherococcus, but lacks the tendency to cause over-excitement that may sometimes occur with ginseng, or constipation as sometimes occurs with eleutherococcus. Russian Rhodiola rosea has been found to be five times less toxic than Panax ginseng [Kelly GS, (2001), Germano, et. al. (1999)].

In many Russian studies, this golden root displayed a significant ability to increase strength and muscle-mass. It was shown to dramatically increase oxygen supply to cells, a requirement for cell growth and regeneration. The herb has been shown to speed recovery from injuries by as much as 100% over normal recovery time. Rhodiola rosea of Russian origin (West and North Siberia) has the highest pharmacological activity and contains the key active components rosavin and salidroside. Interestingly the so-called Tibetan Rhodiola and Rhodiola rosea of Chinese origin very often do not exhibit the same potency.

In one study, the anti-mutagenic activities of Panax ginseng and of Rhodiola rosea were compared. It became clear that the extracts of Rhodiola rosea had a higher capacity to counteract gene mutations induced by various mutagens (up to about 90% inhibition in some cases). Other trials reveal the anti-depressive and anti-stress activity of Rhodiola rosea to be higher than that of St. John's wort, Ginkgo biloba and Panax ginseng.

Controlled studies of Asian ginsengs found improvements in exercise performance when standardized root extracts were used in a study lasting for more than eight weeks, daily dose contained >1 grams of dried root or equivalent. The study groups included a large number of older subjects. Improvements in muscular strength, maximal oxygen uptake, work capacity, fuel homeostasis, heart rate, visual and auditory reaction times, alertness, and psychomotor skills have all been comfortably documented.

Ma huang, ephedrine and related alkaloids have not benefited physical performance except when combined with caffeine. Future research on ergogenic effects of herbs should consider identity and amount of substance or presumed active ingredients administered, dose response, duration of test period, proper experimental controls, measurement of psychological and physiologic parameters (including antioxidant actions) and measurements of performance pertinent to intended uses.

Active Ingredients

There are dozens of substances in Rhodiola rosea, making it difficult to identify which are the active ingredients. Botanists have also identified nearly 200 varieties of Rhodiola rosea. The herb has several unique properties only specific to itself making it quite unique among plants.

Research points out that the most important chemical components that were clinically relevant and specific to Rhodiola rosea species are rosavin, rosin and rosarin. Geraniol was identified as the most important substance responsible for its rose-like odor. Floral notes such as linalool and its oxides, nonanal, decanal, nerol and cinnamyl alcohol highlight the flowery scent of rose root rhizomes. The dried rhizomes contain 0.05% essential oil with the main chemical classes: monoterpene hydrocarbons (25.40%), monoterpene alcohol (23.61%) and straight chain aliphatic alcohol (37.54%). N-Decanol (30.38%), geraniol (12.49%) and 1,4-p-menthadien-7-ol (5.10%) were the most abundant volatiles detected in the essential oil. A total of 86 such compounds have been identified to date.

Molecular structure of Rhodiocyanoside

Recommended Dosage

In Adults: While there appear to be no toxic effects of this herb, high intake is usually well tolerated. The recommended daily maintenance dosage is 100mg to 300mg per day. The therapeutic use of this herb for medical conditions varies, the dosage is usually increased considerably, keeping the toxicity level in mind. This should be undertaken only under the supervision of a knowledgeable herbalist.

In Children, Pregnant and breastfeeding women: It is generally not recommended.

Side Effects and Toxicity

Overall, Rhodiola rosea seems to have very few side effects as it has a very low level of toxicity. In toxicity studies conducted on rats, the lethal dose at which 50 percent of animals die (LD50) was calculated to be 3,360 mg/kg. The equivalent dosage in a 70 kg man would be about 235,000 mg. Since the usual clinical doses are 200-600 mg/day, there is a tremendous margin of safety.

Most individuals who use Rhodiola rosea supplements find that it improves their mood, energy level and mental clarity. Some individuals, particularly those who tend to be anxious, may feel hyperactive, jittery or agitated. If this occurs, then a smaller dose with very gradual increases may be needed.

Several controlled depression studies have found no significant toxicity with the use of this herb. However, at times the body needs to acclimate to new herbal substances. Rhodiola rosea increases serotonin and dopamine levels and reduces cortisol and glucocorticoid levels in persons under stress. The herb does not appear to interact with other medications, although it may have additive effects with other stimulants. It is best absorbed when taken on an empty stomach 30 minutes before breakfast and lunch. Some may want to take Rhodiola rosea early in the day because it can interfere with sleep or cause vivid dreams (not actual nightmares) during the first few weeks of use.

In addition, some trials have found that the following side effects such as irritability, insomnia and unpleasant sensations can occur in some cases in doses above 800mg. No other effects have been observed during clinical trials.

Because Rhodiola rosea has an activating antidepressant effect, it should not be used in individuals with bipolar disorder who are vulnerable to becoming manic when given antidepressants or stimulants. Until this has been further studied, extreme caution should be taken in patients with bipolar spectrum disorders. The herb is also not recommended for persons who suffer nervous excitability, fever or extreme high blood pressure. A final word of caution: As with any herbal preparation, patients should inform their primary healthcare practitioner when taking Rhodiola rosea alone or in any combination.

The Role of Rhodiola rosea in 21st Century Medicine

Although herbs have been used throughout history to enhance physical performance, scientific scrutiny with controlled clinical trials has only recently been used to document the therapeutic effects. Rhodiola rosea of Russian origin is only now becoming more widely accepted in Europe and the USA as a powerful anti-aging, anti-stress supplement. In today's fast-paced culture, this natural herbal remedy may well become an important treatment option in the new science of Longevity Medicine in the 21st Century. This is due in large part to scientific speculation that high stress modern living could well be a main factor causing chronic disease and premature aging as researchers estimate that perhaps as many as 70-80% of all diseases related to aging may occur because of high levels of stress.

As a result, Rhodiola rosea is likely to play an increasing role in both current and future alternative medical applications. Even now, many modern alternative medicine practitioners are prescribing this herbal for combating symptoms like depression, fatigue and stress, as well as to increase longevity and physical endurance. Most importantly, dozens of trials suggest that Rhodiola rosea may help to increase the body's natural resistance to various environmental stressors.

Of course it would be nice to have more scientific research to reaffirm what has already been accomplished to show the preventive and curative benefits of R. rosea. Continued controlled studies are warranted to explore its use in antidepressant augmentation, disorders of memory and cognition, attention deficit disorder, traumatic brain injury, Alzheimer's & Parkinson's disease, sports performance and aviation / space medicine. R. rosea may even have utility in the treatment of heart arrhythmias, infertility, premenstrual disorder, menopause, sexual dysfunction, fibromyalgia, chronic fatigue syndrome, and posttraumatic stress disorder. Enhancement of chemotherapy/radiation with amelioration of toxicity with Rhodiola is another area in medicine justifying exploration.

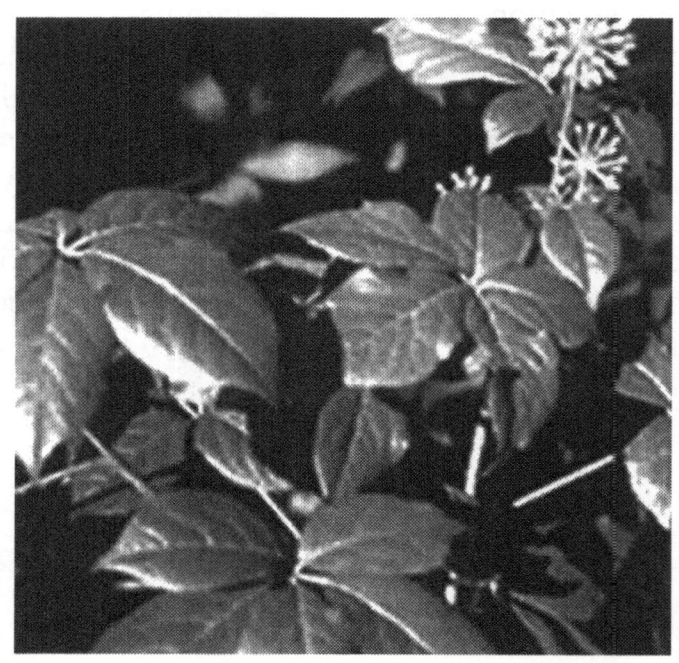

Eleutherococcus senticosus

Chapter II

Eleuthero

By JP Saleeby, MD

Brief History of Eleuthero

E leuthero (Eleutherococcus senticosus) also known by the names Siberian Ginseng, Acanthopanax senticosus, Ci Wu Jia, Devil's Bush, Devil's Shrub, Russian Root, Shigoka, Taiga, Thorny Pepperbush, Touch-me-not, & Wild Pepper is a probably the most familiar adaptogen herbs of the three discussed in this book. After ginseng (Panax ginseng) it reigns second in popularity in the west.

A note on nomenclature before we continue. As we enter a discussion on this important adaptogen herb, it is worth a short aside into the name of this herb. Several historic points prevail relating to the naming of this herb. The confusion may be related in the zeal to find a substitute for the over-harvested P. ginseng in the mid-1900s. During the hunt for a replacement herb for ginseng, Eleuthero was discovered to posses many of the properties of ginseng, therefore it was given the name "Siberian Ginseng".

In 1855 in Russia, two researchers, C. I. Maximovich and L. Shrenk, identified this herb and gave it its current name of genus Eleuthero and species senticocus. It is therefore not of the same genus of Panax ginseng even though it carries many of the same therapeutic effects. The distinguishing factor of Eleuthero is its woody and twisted root. This is what differentiates it from P. ginseng. The term "seng" in Chinese refers to that of a "fleshy rootstock" by those Chinese herbologists who describe the true ginseng roots which have this characteristic. Eleuthero does not meet either the physical phytotaxonomical or phytogeographical characteristics and should not be classified as a "ginseng". Additionally in 2002 the United States Farm Security and Rural Investment Act made it illegal to use the name "ginseng" for any product not derived from the genus Panax. Consequently the nomenclature "Siberian Ginseng" is really a misnomer and should not be used.

The plant is a spiny shrub in the family Araliaceae and grows to be approx 9 to 10 feet in height. Erect shoots are about an inch or more in diameter. It has a darkish-brown bark which is thickly covered with small pale thorns or bristles that point downward. The leaves are grouped in 5 leaflets that are elliptic and finely serrated. As with ginseng, the roots are usually harvested in the fall and the leaves and branches are harvested before it flowers in mid-summer.

This herb is found commonly in East Asia (China, Japan, Korea and Siberia). It tends to grow in mixed coniferous mountain forests. In the Western Hemisphere it is found in Oregon and Montana. Originally harvested in the wild, this herb is now cultivated worldwide. Much like P. ginseng, over-harvesting of Eleuthero in the wild has lead to near extinction of this herb in some regions and therefore this herb is now grown commercially.

Eleuthero is consumed in many forms. From standardized tablets and capsules to the chewing of boiled roots, to teas, infusions and tinctures (33% ethanol extract). However, it was reported that a rather useful polysaccharide involved in immune boosting may precipitate out of alcohol extracts of the root. So care is needed in deciding which preparation is to be used for what ailment. Read labels carefully and make sure the nomenclature is specific and correct. A common adulterant found in some Eleuthero products is Periploca sepium.

There is a case-study which identified the adulterant P. sepium as the actual culprit in an adverse reaction that was blamed on Eleuthero. The study was reported in JAMA in 1990 (Koren, et. al.) where a neonate suffered androgenization due to maternal use of "Eleuthero". However, follow up studies by Awang, et. al. (1991) and Waller, et. al. (1992) showed no signs of androgenicity and conclude that the culprit herb was the contaminant P. sepium, and in fact held harmless Eleuthero.

Storing raw herbs, tinctures or teas in airtight containers between 15 and 30oC is imperative for longevity of potency. For practicality it is best to purchase standardized preparations in capsule or tablet form.

How Eleuthero is used

Eleuthero is used to treat a wide variety of diseases. According to research, this adaptogen has actions stronger than those of P. ginseng and is thought to improve cognitive function and increase longevity [Winther K, et al (1997)]. It is used to increase stamina and boost the immune system [Williams M, (1995)]. Traditional Chinese Medicine (TCM) has used it as a remedy for insomnia and for those in stress or stressful situations. TCM uses this adaptogen herb to reinforce Qi and invigorate the function of the spleen and kidneys referred to as yang deficiency. In a report from Duke & Ayensu (1985) Eleuthero was reported to be used in Harbin, China as a folk medicine remedy for heart ailments, bronchitis and rheumatic disease.

Reducing Stress and Fatigue

Eleuthero is reported to have utility in restoring general health, vigor, memory, promoting appetite and increasing longevity. Russian research in the 1950's and 60's led scientists such as Dr. Israel I. Brekhman (a highly regarded herbologist on Eleuthero) to publish work reporting it as a true adaptogen herb and showing no evidence of toxicity. In Russia, Eleuthero is widely used in their deep sea divers, cosmonauts and athletes as well as mountain rescue workers, explorers, soldiers and factory workers for its stated restorative and stamina properties. In Germany, the government approves Eleuthero for use in treating the fatigued and debilitated as reported by Blumenthal (1996).

A well-known study conducted in 1985 by Farnsworth showed many beneficial effects of this primary adaptogen herb. The reported benefits include increased alertness, increased work output and increased quality of work under stressful conditions in normal human volunteers as well as in athletes.

In the Soviet Union when productivity was a measure of the regimes health, adaptogens were studied intently as a means to keep the working class health, enhance stamina and recuperate them from illness. Thus there was much research on this herb for the general populous. Large populations of workers under clinical study were shown to have a decrease between 30 and 35% in disease incidence. In a study of miners over a two-month period illness reported a drop by 33.3% and days missed from work dropped by 45.6%. When Eleuthero was compared with placebo in respiratory infections in a mining study group it lessened the incidence of disease 2.4 fold. This herb enhances stamina and physical performance (and athletic performance) by supporting the adrenal glands during chronic bouts of stress, environmental toxins and drug (including caffeine) use or abuse.

Many people today are overwhelmed by stress and fatigue, which results in adrenal gland dysfunction. Stress has weighs heavy on the Hypothalamus-Pituitary-Adrenal (HPA) axis or system. For a diagram of this neuro-endocrine system see Table 2 in the Appendix. Today fatigue and stress are growing complaints doctors are hearing from their patients. Dr. Hans Selye (1907-1982) was an internationally renown "stress" researcher and coined the term General Adaptation Syndrome. This syndrome has three stages: Alarm Reaction, Adaptation and Exhaustion. In the alarm reaction stage the body detects the external stressful stimuli. The adaptation stage results in the bodies engaging in defensive countermeasures against the stress stimulus. Finally in the exhaustion stage the body begins to run out of its defenses, and fatigue sets in. In Japan, where stress and competitiveness are extremely high in the workplace, they have a term for "death from overworking" called karoshi, the result of high levels of stress causing heart attack and stroke. Adaptogen herbs play a significant role in preventing disease in all of Selye's stages of stress [Hiai S. et. al. (1979), Fulder S, (1981)]. They are especially useful in the adaptation stage as the name signifies and also in the exhaustion stage to help ward off fatigue and support and extend adrenal function.

Adrenal gland dysfunction can be the root cause of such symptoms as fatigue, weakness, feelings of being run down, metabolic disturbances, immune system problems and thyroid gland disturbances. Constant stress (both physical and emotional), disorders such as Cushing's syndrome and Addison's disease, as well as poor nutrition are ways a person can succumb to disruption of proper adrenal gland function.

The adrenal glands lay just anterior-superior to both kidneys and are responsible for production and secretion of special steroidal and peptide hormones. Despite their relative small size they are non-the-less very important glands. The hormones responsible for maintaining blood pressure and acting as excitatory neurotransmitters are produced from the inner most part of the gland called the medulla. The outer aspect (cortex) secretes other classes of compounds called steroid hormones, which are all important in maintaining good health.

The adrenal gland hormones play a critical role in human immune function and maintaining a balance of serum electrolytes, such as sodium and potassium. Disturbance of this gland's function can have a profound impact on a person's health, while total shut down or suppression of the gland can result in severe morbidity and even death. Adaptogen herbs are a natural way to support this important gland.

Bolstering the Immune System

Research has shown Eleuthero's immune system bolstering is due to stimulation of T-cell production. Eleuthero has the ability to improve blood lipids, is considered an antioxidant, acts as a vasodilator and anti-inflammatory and reduces elevated blood glucose levels. A three-month human study showed this adaptogen helpful in memory and concentration when compared with a placebo. When this herb was studied in those afflicted with viral infections results varied. However, Eleuthero slowed the replication of the Influenza-A virus, human rhinovirus and respiratory syncytial virus (RSV) in one study. While it had no effect on adenovirus or herpes simplex type-1, it did reduce frequency, severity and duration of herpes simplex type-2 viral outbreaks in a 6-month study of 93 people. Drs. Wagner & Proksch (1985) were able to report immuno-potentiating effects in immune cells. They found that Eleuthero enhanced the action of phagocyte cells in a process called phagocytosis, as well as enhancing adjuvant activity in B-lymphocytes.

While in theory Eleuthero may be helpful during the cold and flu season, there are few trials to substantiate its effects. However in healthy people taking 10 ml of a standardized tincture three times a day it was shown to increase the number of T4-lymphocytes. Since T4-lymphocytes are depressed in HIV and AIDs patients, this herb may find utility in their treatment [Glatthaar-Saalmuller B, et. al (2001)]. Further research is needed in this field.

Other Benefits of Eleuthero

Research has shown this adaptogen helpful in the treatment and prevention of neuroses, coronary artery disease, diabetes, hypertension, bronchitis, cancers, acute head injury, combating radiation sickness and toxic chemical exposures. During the days that followed the horrific Chernobyl nuclear accident, many Russian and Ukrainian citizens were given Eleuthero to counter the effects of the radioactive fallout. This herbs effects were actually well documented by researchers in in vitro laboratory studies for use in radiation sickness.

Studies suggest that this herb may be helpful in alleviating side effects and bone marrow suppression in people undergoing radiation therapy and chemotherapy for the treatment of cancers. However, always consult your oncologist before taking this herb in conjunction with cancer therapies.

Active Ingredients

The active ingredients in Eleuthero are knows as eleuthero-sides. There are seven primary eleutherosides that have been identified by scientists. Most research has been focused on eleutherosides B and E. Eleuthero also contains complex polysaccharide molecules and they may be critical players in the role of this herb on the support of the immune system.

R1	OCH3
R2	O-β-D-Glc
R3	OCH3
R4	OCH3
R5	O-β-D-Glc
R6	OCH3

Molecular structure of a Eleutheroside

Usual Doses

Generally recommended adults doses are as follows. When taking the dried root to be chewed after boiling or in the form of a tea or infusion, a dose of 500 mg to 3000 mg (3g) daily is recommended. Low dose is considered 1.0 to 2.0 grams per day while high dose is 9.0 to 15.0 grams per day. The average dose is usually between 2.0 to 6.0 grams daily. With regards to Tinctures (in alcohol) a dose of 1 teaspoon three times a day is recommended. Fluid extract (1:1) 1/2 to 1 tsp. two to three times a day, and extracts in alcohol (33%) 40 to 120 drops one to three times daily.

Probably the most practical and recommended form is the solid tablet / capsule formulation. Solid extracts made from dried or powdered root containing standardized 1% eleutheroside are taken in 100mg to 200mg doses three times a day.

In pediatric patients it is not generally recommended due to the herbs stimulant effects. When used by an experienced practitioner it should be limited to no more than 2 consecutive weeks in a mild or low dose regiment. In pregnant and nursing females it is used with caution.

Duration of therapy for most conditions should be cycled. The most typical cycle is one month on the adaptogen herb and one month off. For more severe chronic conditions it can be safely taken for three months followed by a 2 to 3-week "herbal holiday". These cycles can be repeated indefinitely under the direction of a medical practitioner.

Side Effects and Toxicity

Since Eleuthero is a much more common herb in the West, it has been under scrutiny for a longer period of time, thus more reported toxicity and side effects have been documented. This has not been the case with Jiaogulan and Rhodiola rosea. It should be noted that those with uncontrolled hypertension should be cautious with this herb. Also those who are pregnant, nursing mothers and children should use this herb carefully. Those with obstructive sleep apnea should avoid this herb, as should those with narcolepsy. Caution should be taken with large doses of Eleuthero in diabetic patients, as this herb can reduce the serum glucose levels and cause hypoglycemia. If it is used in a diabetic, careful blood glucose monitoring should be conducted while on the herb.

Side effects are listed as headaches, insomnia (rare), anxiety, irritability, breast pain, and drowsiness. Other lesser symptoms include irregular heart rhythm, nosebleeds and vomiting. To prevent insomnia the herb should not be taken less than six hours before bedtime. There are reported cases of changes in the taste of certain spicy or bitter foods while taking Eleuthero.

There may be interactions with other medications and herbs. Due to inhibition of metabolic breakdown there is a concern of interaction with hexobarbital resulting in an increased effect [Medon et. al (1984)]. Eleuthero also interacts with antibiotics increasing their effectiveness by enhancing T-lymphocyte activity. This drug-herb interaction may not necessarily be a bad thing.

When Eleuthero is taken with Lanoxin® (digoxin) it has been shown in several studies [McRae (1996), Miller (1998)] to raise blood levels. So caution must be taken when taking this herb and digoxin concomitantly. If it is necessary, serum digoxin levels should be closely monitored. Eleuthero has been shown to increase the clotting time of blood. When taken with anticoagulant drugs such as heparin or warfaran or antiplatelet drugs such as aspirin or Plavix®, uncontrolled bleeding is a risk.

Caution should be taken when used in combination with glucose lowering drugs such as Actos®, Amaryl®, Avandia®, Glucotrol®, Glynase®, Glucophage®, Prandin®, Precose®

and the hormone Insulin. Symptomatic hypoglycemia may be noted. If Eleuthero is to be a regular part of a diabetics regiment it can be used to lower the doses of hypoglycemic agents and exogenous insulin demand, but only under strict supervision of a knowledgeable physician.

Increased sleep is a consequence of use with carbamazepine, phenytoin, valproic acid, barbiturates, benzodiazepines and sleeping aids such as Ambien®, Sonata® and other sleep aids. Eleuthero can also increase sleepiness when used with tricyclic antidepressants (TCA) such as amitriptyline, doxepin and nortriptyline. Over the counter drugs like diphenhydramine and alcoholic beverages are not immune here. This has to do with how the body metabolizes these drugs when Eleuthero on board.

As Dr. G. Henderson et. al. (1999) demonstrated, Eleuthero interferes with the same enzyme pathway (cytocrome P450 system) that breaks down some drugs, thus the following should be used with caution. Drugs like the antihistamine Allegra®, and anti-fungals Nizoral® and Sporanox® can have their pharmokenetics changed. Cancer drugs such as etoposide, paclitaxel and vinblastine also clear differently. The muscle relaxant Flexeril® and the cholesterol drugs Lovastatin® are a couple of drugs affected by this herb. Also use with caution with the drugs fluvoxamine, Haldol®, birth control pills, and theophylline as metabolism may be diminished and levels may rise.

Some herbal interactions include inhibiting of blood clotting with Danshen, Devil's Claw, garlic, ginger, ginkgo, horse chestnut, Panax Ginseng, papain, red clover, and saw palmetto. Hypoglycemia can occur when used in combination with fenugreek, ginger, kudzu, and p. ginseng. Sedating effects are seen with use in conjunction with catnip, hops, Kava, St. John's wort, and Valerian root.

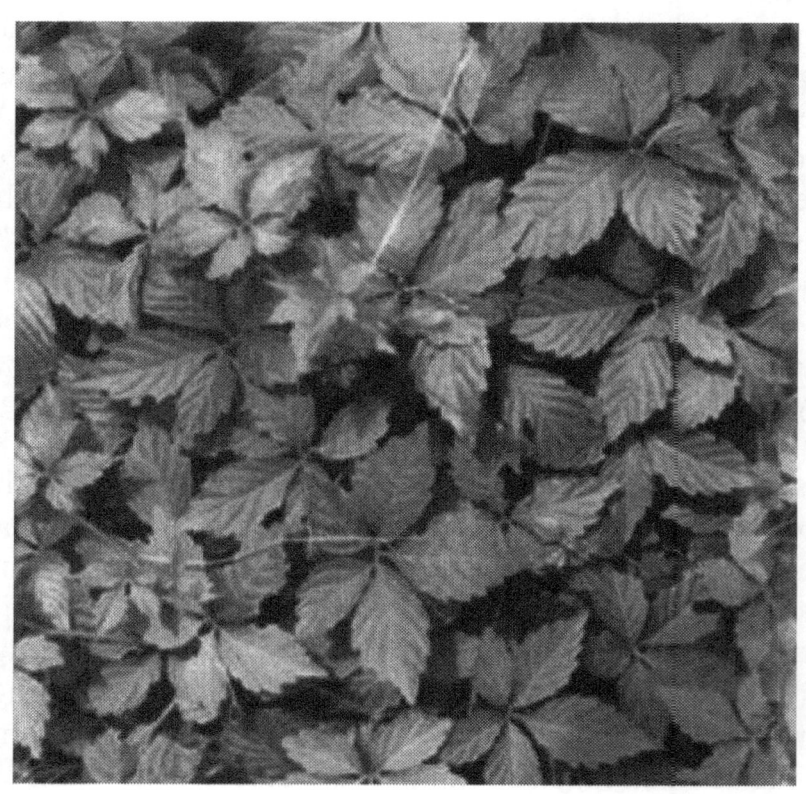

Gynostemma pentaphyllum

Chapter III

Jiaogulan

JP Saleeby, M.D. and Amber P. Keefer

Brief History of Jiaogulan

Most of us are familiar with the wide-ranging medicinal uses of ginseng, but a little-known Asian herb is slowly gaining market share and becoming a popular herbal supplement on today's growing market of alternative therapies. Reputed to boost the immune system, this herbal Adaptogen is being used to treat everything from high blood pressure to insomnia.

Jiaogulan (Gynostemma pentaphyllum), less commonly known as Jagulana, or the 'Five-Leaf Ginseng', is a plant that grows wild in the mountains of southern China. A member of the gourd family, the herb can also be found in Japan, Korea and India. Sometimes called Southern Ginseng), Jiaogulan, pronounced (gee-OW-goolahn), has been commonly used as a tonic and medicinal herb in the Oriental regions where it has grown since the 16th century. Because of its many therapeutic qualities and reputation for preventing the signs of aging, the Chinese call it the 'immortality herb'. It's first documented use and discovery can be seen in the recordings and sketch of the plant in Zhu Xiao's book Materia Medica for Famine in 1406 A.D. around the time of the beginning of the Ming Dynasty. In the years that followed during the Qing dynasty (1644-1912 A.D.) an herbalist named Wu Qi-Jun in his text Textual Investigation of Herbal Plants further classified the herb dispelling some confusion this Adaptogen herb had with another named Wulianmei.

The reason for this fascinating herb not being more commonly prescribed is in fact a matter of geography. Jiaogulan grows in the more mountainous regions of southern China far from the bed of ancient Chinese herbology referred to as the "ancient domain of China." This ancient domain is located more in the center of the country. The system we refer today as Traditional Chinese Medicine (TCM) has its birthplace in this ancient domain. So Jiaogulan growing predominantly in a region far from most herbs harvested by TCM practitioners took a back seat to some of the more commonly seen and grown herbs of the day. However, the more worldly or experienced herbologist has used this herb as it is cited in several texts as being something that enhances "Yin" and supports "Yang". It has been used traditionally to treat hematuria, edema, pain of the pharynx, swelling of the neck, tumors and even trauma. This herb is used to increase the resistance to infection and for its inflammatory fighting properties.

In fact, rumor has it that once when the Chinese were performing a census, they found one province with the most centenarians (people living over hundred years old). When officials looked into the differences between the people of that province and others, they found that they were drinking Jiaogulan as a tea. Thus the term "Immortality Herb" or Xiancao, by the locals, stuck.

Jiaogulan, which has been extensively researched in both China and Japan for the past two decades, has been found to contain a variety of saponins known as gypenosides—plant chemicals similar in structure to human steroid hormones.

The Japanese refer to this herb as Amachazuru, the components of this word meaning "Amacha" (sweet)—"cha" (tea) and "zuru" (vine). Other names in use for this herb are Miracle Grass, Southern Ginseng, Vitis Pentaphyllum and Xianxao (Immortal Herb).

Although the extract from the leaves of this plant has been used for healing purposes in the southeastern provinces of China for centuries, it wasn't until recently that Jiaogulan has been introduced in the U.S. However, the herb is getting a lot of attention these days as the scientific community takes a closer interest in how these plant chemicals can benefit human health and performance. Awareness in the herb's health-enhancing qualities was sparked, when in the late 1970's, Dr. Osama Tanaka [(Takemoto (1984)] a Japanese researcher, looking for a sugar alternative, studied a perennial weed known for its sweetness. What he discovered was an herb with many qualities similar to ginseng in chemical composition and action. Clinical research in 1972 yielded a study with reported benefits in 537 case subjects with chronic tracheo-bronchitis [Qu, J. (1972)].

Since then, scientists around the world have conducted several clinical studies on the therapeutic effectiveness of gypenosides. As a result, a number of scientifically controlled studies have found that Jiaogulan is an effective adaptogen, as well as a potent antioxidant. The herb was also found to contain trace minerals, amino acids, proteins and vitamins, substances all vital to overall health and well-being.

The results of extensive laboratory, animal and human research in recent years have shown Jiaogulan to have many beneficial, preventive and therapeutic effects. Traditionally brewed as a tea, many products are now being made from the extract of Jiaogulan, either as a single herb supplement or in combination with other Chinese herbs.

Jiaogulan is a perennial vine and unlike it's ginseng counterpart it is a much faster growing herb. This vine grows very rapidly in the warm climates at a rate documented as two and a half inches a day. The vine has leaves that divide into five leaflets. The largest leaflet is usually at the end of the stem. While this plant is in the same family as the cucumbers, zucchini and melons it does not bear any edible fruit, but instead a small dark berry. The berry is the product of a small light yellow flower. The seeds will sprout new plants but the main way this plant spreads is by producing new shoots from it underground runner roots. This plant is harvest in late summer [Zhu, X, et. al., (1990)]. The herb is very well cultivated for commercial use because of its heartiness and quick growth.

How Jiaogulan is used

Jiaogula is an adaptogenic herb and by definition it helps the body to adjust or resist stress. Adaptogens recharge the adrenal glands, which are the body's normal mechanism for responding to stress and emotional changes.

Studies suggest that Jiaogulan regulates the body's nervous and hormonal systems when they are adversely affected by stress. Put more simply, Jiaogulan helps put back into balance what is "out of whack!" According to recent studies, the herb contains nearly four times as many saponins as Panax ginseng. Dr. Takemoto, a Jiaogulan researcher, discovered four saponins that are shared with Panax ginseng. But all in all there have been identified eighty-two saponins where Panax has only twenty-eight. So we have an almost four-fold greater number of saponins in Jiaogulan. Saponins are unusual substances due to their physical properties that allow them to dissolve in both water and lipids (oils). Researchers are in agreement that the saponins are probably the more active components in these medicinal herbs.

A large body of medical research in the past few years has shown that this adaptogenic herbal aids in regulating cholesterol and blood pressure, reduces blood sugar and strengthens the immune system. It has also been shown to improve circulation and cardiovascular function, increase stamina, reduce stress, stimulate liver function and promote restful sleep. Mice tested in the laboratory show without a doubt the benefits of Jiaogulan in endurance, anti-cancer and positive adaptogenic effects that counteract the untoward effects of steroids (corticosteroids) [Arichi, S. et. al. (1985)]. Nearly 300 scientific papers on Jiaogulan and its saponins have been published in respected scientific journals.

Regulation of Blood Pressure

It's no secret that problems with either high or low blood pressure can cause many health problems, sometimes even leading to serious complications. A number of studies have shown that Jiaogulan controls blood pressure by lowering it when it is too high or raising it when it is too low.

One study illustrated that by taking 300 mg of Jiaogulan regularly one can reduce high blood pressure in just weeks. The mechanism of action is by increasing production of nitric oxide, a chemical that relaxes blood vessel walls. In another research trial, the effectiveness for a group of patients taking Jiaogulan was rated nearly as high as the group taking prescribed blood pressure medication.

Researchers have also concluded that Jiaogulan helps to regulate blood pressure by increasing blood circulation and decreasing resistance in blood vessels. For this very reason this herb is regarded as rather effective in the treatment of hypertension.

In a clinical trial of patients suffering from hypertension, the effect of Jiaogulan were compared with that of ginseng. The results revealed that 82 percent of those taking Jiaogulan noted improvement in their condition as opposed to only 46 percent of those patients taking ginseng.

Regulation of Blood Lipids

Numerous trials [Lin C, et. al. (2001), Kang J, et. al. (2000)] have found that Jiaogulan helps maintain normal cholesterol levels by improving the ratio of HDL (high-density lipoprotein)—good cholesterol—to LDL (low-density lipoprotein)—bad cholesterol. Published reports show that jiaogulan can dramatically lower blood serum levels of total cholesterol, phospholipids and dangerous LDL cholesterol, while increasing beneficial HDL cholesterol.

Jiaogulan is thought to increase lipid metabolism, which includes the conversion of cholesterol to Vitamin D, bile acid and HDL. It also inhibits the production of free fatty acids, which leads to triglyceride synthesis by the body's fat cells. In lowering the LDL cholesterol, Jiaogulan can help prevent atherosclerosis, stroke and heart attack. Likewise, increasing levels of HDL removes excess cholesterol as waste and helps protect cells from damage caused by low-density lipoproteins.

Clinical data suggests that Jiaogulan decreases cholesterol by improving the liver's ability to send sugar and carbohydrates to the muscles for conversion to energy instead of turning the sugar into triglycerides that the body stores as fat. In a number of studies, the effectiveness of treatment using gypenosides to lower total cholesterol was shown to be as much as 63 percent.

Jiaogulan also appears to improve fat metabolism and increase the absorption of nutrients. It appears to also block the absorption of fat, depress lipid peroxide and fat sediment in the blood vessels.

Improving Circulation and Cardiovascular Function

Research indicates that Jiaogulan increases the efficiency of the heart's pumping mechanism. In other words, it helps the heart pump the same amount of blood with less effort and stress. And when the heart doesn't have to work as hard, it remains stronger and more efficient. In point of fact, in one animal study, the use of gypenosides was shown to considerably reduce the damage from heart attack [Purmova J, et. al. (1995)]

By increasing the body's blood supply through enhanced cardiac output, Jiaogulan helps to nourish the internal organs by getting more oxygen to cells. Since oxygen plays a pivotal role in cellular metabolism and activity, more oxygen means greater endurance and increased stamina. Jiaogulan also contributes to a healthier heart because of its capacity to help the body cope with the harmful effects of stress, which can be a major element in the development of heart disease. Incidentally, improved cardiac output has been shown to shorten recovery time from illness and injury.

One trial studied 220 athletes as well as 30 healthy non-athletes taking Jiaogulan and showed a significant increase in cardiac output via ultrasound color doppler (ECHO) examination. This was achieved without an increase in blood pressure or pulse rate.

Jiaogulan seems to be effective as a general cardiovascular enhancer as gypenosides from the herb promote the release of nitric acid from vascular tissue, which helps to relax the coronary blood vessels thus widening the blood vessel lumen and increase circulation.

Other studies indicate that the herb may help maintain the normal viscosity of the blood. Subcutaneous injection of 50mg Jiaogulan gypenosides resulted in inhibiting the development of atherosclerosis in experimental rats in a study by Dr. G. Qi et. al. (2000). The rate of platelet thrombosis was 34 percent lower than those of the test animals in control groups.

Similarly, rats receiving 35mg of Jiaogulan extract intravenously for 10-20 minutes showed an inhibition of platelet aggregation. Platelet aggregation, which is associated with atherosclerosis, stroke and heart attack, is the basis for formation of blood clots [Tan (1993)]. Therefore, the ability of Jiaogulan to inhibit platelet aggregation and prevent plaque buildup can reduce the chance for both atherosclerosis and coronary heart disease.

Boosting the Immune System

Clinical research studies indicate that Jiaogulan is effective at helping the body resist depression of the immune system and may increase the production of white blood cells in patients who have recently undergone chemotherapy or radiation treatments. This herbal was also found to improve the Natural Killer (NK) cell activity in cancer patients, thereby helping their bodies to fight back against the invading tumors.

Jiaogulan strengthens the immune system by preventing stress hormones that weaken immunity from overpowering the body, making a person more vulnerable to illness. When the body is under stress, humans produces hormones. These hormones sometimes over-stimulate the nervous system and trigger more stress hormones, a snow balling effect that healthy individuals want to eliminate.

Research suggests that a daily dose of Jiaogulan could lessen the risk of colds, flu and infections by increasing the production of infection-fighting blood cells. In one controlled study, young rats fed with jiaogulan extract showed an increase in the number of T-lymphocytes. In addition, results of data collected from an animal model heart transplant showed that gypenosides infusion can reduce the risk of host rejection, caused by immuno-incompatibility, to a transplanted organ. Another example of the bi-directionality of adaptogen herbs.

Support of Liver Function

A number of studies [Lin, J (2000), & Chen JC (1999)] show that Jiaogulan may produce anti-inflammatory effects that protect the liver from various toxic chemicals such as carbon tetrachloride. Jiaogulan (50mg daily) was shown to activate DNA replication in liver cells, thus promoting liver regeneration.

In Taiwan, the herb is used to treat liver disease and to protect liver tissue from damage as the gypenosides found in Jiaogulan have been shown to have a protective effect on liver cells. In fact, researchers who recently studied the herbal for its effect on liver disease reported that Jiaogulan significantly improves recovery from liver injury and prevents development of liver fibrosis.

A Chinese study showed that patients with chronic hepatitis B treated with gypenosides for 3 months obtained satisfactory improvement in hepatic function.

Lowering Blood Glucose

Along with all its other therapeutic uses, Jiaogulan is now being promoted as a supplement for natural glucose balance. Medical studies indicate that gypenosides in the herb suppress the absorption of glucose in the intestinal tract, thus lowering blood sugar levels.

Clinical studies in lab animals show that Jiaogulan extract appears to stimulate rejuvenation of essential pancreatic Beta cells, the key cell responsible in the generation of insulin. Findings indicate that the hypoglycemic activity of Jiaogulan is due to its ability to stimulate insulin release from the pancreas. Results from a glucose tolerance test suggest that extract from the herb may also exhibit an inhibitory effect on glucose absorption and reduce the metabolic effects of sugar by preventing the intestines from absorbing the sugar molecules during the process of digestion.

Controlled studies of gypenosides on glucose metabolism using both animal and human models reveal that gypenosides effectively reduce blood glucose level in animals and patients with diabetes mellitus. Jiaogulan extract (200mg) added to food or 100mg IV for 3 days was shown to reduce the blood glucose level in insulin-dependent diabetic mice. Another animal study used gypenosides to treat rats with diabetes mellitus for four weeks and found that the blood glucose, insulin, triglycerides and total cholesterol were lowered markedly.

One human clinical trial used gypenosides to treat 46 patients with diabetes mellitus for eight weeks. Results showed that the herb lowered blood glucose. Glycohemoglobin, cholesterol, triglycerides, LDL and blood viscosity were also lowered to the normal range, whereas serum HDL increased with treatment.

Gypenosides were used to treat 80 patients with type-2 diabetes mellitus with satisfactory results—decreased serum insulin and blood glucose levels. Since insulin resistance and impaired glucose tolerance characterize Type II diabetes, it appears that the gypenosides found in jiaogulan can increase insulin sensitivity in diabetics, even in patients without high lipid levels. It can even reduce the symptoms of associated with glycosuria (sugar in the urine).

Enhancing Athletic Performance

Jiaogulan can be used as a safe and legal ergogenic aid in sports. A study of 300 athletes testing Jiaogulan (taken prior to competition versus a control group given placebo) yielded results that showed increased alertness, quicker reflexes and less nervousness with increased vigor only in test subjects taking the adaptogen herb.

Avoiding the Signs of Aging

Who doesn't want to avoid the signs of aging? But oxidative damage to cells caused by free radicals—unstable oxygen molecules generated in the body as by-products of metabolism—can damage or destroy healthy cells. The bad news is the damage to cells and tissues produced by these free radicals can accelerate the aging processes.

Even though the body needs free radicals to function properly, (i.e. when the body is attacked by an invading virus, white blood cells generate free radicals to deactivate foreign micro-organisms), they can become a problem when there are too many of them. It may help to understand that when a cell undergoes oxidation, it loses electrons, which affects its chemical composition. But when oxygen molecules lose electrons, free radicals will search the body for another cell, affecting its structure and function. In the meantime, these unpaired, unstable electrons can wreak havoc on any one of the body's systems as they try to pair with other electrons. As unstable oxygen molecules are produced (not only by the body's functions and metabolism, but also by environmental factors such as radiation, cigarette smoke, pollution and alcohol) they do damage to our organ systems. The fight against free radicals is a tough and complex battle.

The good news is that research studies show Jiaogulan can prolong the life span of cells by strengthening cellular functions and promoting cell proliferation. The herb also lowers the amount of superoxide radicals and hydrogen peroxide in certain white blood cells. Researchers have indicated that the active elements of Jiaogulan actually scavenge the body for these free radicals. In doing so, they protect the body from DNA damage caused by oxidation and ward off the inevitable physical signs of aging.

Jiaogulan works by increasing levels of the body's naturally occurring antioxidant, superoxide dismutase (SOD), who's job it is to protect cells from oxidative damage [Zhou, S, (1990)]. And that can translate into fewer wrinkles. SOD cannot be taken as an oral supplement. It is too fragile a substance to withstand our gastrointestinal system. One viable alternative is oral Jiaogulan, but there remain others as well.

Scientific studies illustrate that taking 40mg of Jiaogulan daily can triple the body's production of superoxide dismutase, thereby helping to neutralize damaging free radicals. Among 106 people in one trial taking Jiaogulan gypenosides (40mg/capsule), 2 capsules 3 times a day for 2 months, more than 80 percent reported improvement in kidney and spleen functions, physical strength and the relief of backache and insomnia.

According to researchers, there is growing evidence that free radical damage caused by oxidation of cell membrane lipids may be reduced by the widespread antioxidant effect of gypenosides found in Jiaogulan and may aid in the prevention and treatment of degenerative diseases like cancer, cataracts, atherosclerosis and liver disease that are all associated with aging.

Through animal testing, scientists found that gypenosides protected the experimental animals from various kinds of oxidative damage, which was induced by introduction of free radicals. Good correlation was found between delaying of the aging process and the reduction of free radical damage.

A clinical study of 610 healthy persons, 50-90 years of age, found that with the increase of age, SOD decreased. However, following oral administration of 20mg of gypenosides twice daily for one month, a significant increase in the serum SOD level was reported in the 50-69 year-old group. The results of this study showed that gypenosides can induce endogenous production of SOD.

Other studies indicate that by decreasing oxidative DNA damage and cell division, anti-oxidants like Jiaogulan may help the body defend itself against degenerative diseases. Jiaogulan may also act as an anti-carcinogen, and thus help reduce the risk of cancer. This is important because most cancer risk increases with age and our aging population may benefit from the routine use of this herb.

Reducing the Risk of Cancer

Because of its strong antioxidant effect, Jiaogulan is believed to obstruct the growth of cancer [Arichi et. al.

(1985)]. In vitro (test tube) experimental studies have shown Jiaogulan gypenosides to inhibit tumor growth of cancers of the stomach, rectum, breast, uterus, oral cavity, liver, brain, lung, kidney, tongue, thymus, thyroid, prostate and skin. Jiaogulan also appears able to slow down melanoma proliferation.

In an animal study, a test group of rats was given Jiaogulan two weeks prior to the introduction of a carcinogen. After 18 weeks of receiving the carcinogen, not only did researchers observe that the number of tumors in the test group was lower than those in the group that received only the carcinogen, they noted that Jiaogulan might actually have delayed the onset of the cancer for six weeks. The mechanism of action for anticancer properties is the increase in Natural Killer (NK) cell activity.

It should be noted, however, that the effect of Jiaogulan on cancer is still in the experimental stage. Although animal studies have confirmed Jiaogulan as an inhibitor or retarder of the growth of malignant tumor induced by application of a carcinogen, its effect on inhibiting various types of human cancer cells in the human model warrants further investigation.

Other Benefits o Jiaogulan

Chinese have traditionally used Jiaogulan for decades in curing bronchitis and other respiratory ailments [Qu, J, (1972)]. Historically, extract from the herb has been used to treat bronchitis, coughs and infectious hepatitis.

Recent studies report that in 86 cases of chronic bronchitis, the effectiveness rate of Jiaogulan tea was 93 percent. Another study cited a 92 percent effectiveness rate in 96 cases of chronic bronchitis. Tests show that Jiaogulan acts as a natural sedative and has been found to be effective in promoting and improving the overall quality of sleep.

In addition, it has been reported that Jiaogulan gypenosides, supplemented with ethanol, peppermint and glycerol, could prevent hair loss and gray hair. Treatment of 1g/day for 3 months has also been shown to improve capillary blood circulation and promote hair growth. One report also indicates that the mixture of Jiaogulan gypenosides and Vitamin C taken orally can prevent the unpleasant body odor found with perspiration.

In studies involving a group of thrombocytopenia (a decrease in the number of blood platelets) patients, Jiaogulan treatment (40mg/dose, 3 doses/day for 1 month) revealed a significant increase in the number of platelets in the blood. As mentioned previously Chinese studies have even found Jiaogulan to reduce blood clots in human blood [Tan, H, et. al. (1993)].

Jiaogulan extract of 40-50 percent has been reported to slow down various degrees of bacterial infection, especially in the respiratory and gastrointestinal tracts. There are those researchers who believe that Jiaogulan can elevate the rate of protein synthesis in organ tissues like spleen, testis, cerebrum and the blood circulatory system. This herb may even play a role in weight-loss by curbing appetite and increasing the sense of fullness.

Active Ingredients

The chemical makeup of these gypenosides resembles ginsenosides, the active ingredients of ginseng. Jiaogulan contains 82 distinct gypenosides, four times the number of different saponins found in ginseng, making it a more complex and possibly more significant adaptogen [Yoshikawa (1987)].

Molecular structure of a gypenoside

Usual doses

A typical dose of Jiaogulan is 1,000mg per day in the form of tea or in capsules, but much higher doses appear to be safe and effective. Standardized extracts should provide a dose containing 25-200mg of gypenosides per day.

Studies indicate that 300mg daily may cut artery-clogging LDL-cholesterol levels by as much as 25 percent. And when it comes to suppressing the free radicals that cause the signs of aging, clinical trials show that taking 40mg of Jiaogulan daily increases production of the chemical, superoxide dismutase, thereby neutralizing free radicals.

For those who can't sleep because of stress, a supplement of just 80mg of Jiaogulan daily may have you sleeping better with a week. Preliminary research suggests Jiaogulan boosts infection-fighting blood cells so dramatically that just

240mg taken daily could cut cancer-cell production by 30 percent. Three doses of Jiaogulan extract daily, (each dose of 2grams), for 30-40 days was confirmed to significantly lower blood pressure, myocardial infarction and kidney disease with up to 88 percent effectiveness.

Unfortunately the standardization of this herb is difficult. Depending on the species and conditions of growth and harvesting there is wide variability in the concentrations of the some 80 different saponins in this herb. While the FDA does not require nor regulate herbal standardizations, the products available in the market place can reach both ends of the continuum of quality and strength. So research your product choice well. Again this herb is not generally recommended for the pediatric, pregnant or breastfeeding population.

Side Effects and Toxicity

Very few reported adverse side effects have been seen with Jiaogulan to date. It should be noted that for cardiac patients, Jiaogulan does not appear to have the over-stimulating effects that ginseng sometimes causes. Some accounts of nausea with an increase in number of bowel movements daily is reported with high doses.

Like any prescription drug, herbal remedies should be taken with caution. It is important to make your physician aware if you are taking herbal supplements, especially if you are currently taking prescription medications simultaneously.

Jiaogulan (or many other herbal remedies for that matter) is not generally recommended for use by pregnant women, those women trying to become pregnant or those breastfeeding. Animal studies show some birth defects with gynostemma use, but no human studies are around to report similar effects. It is therefore agreed that pregnant mothers should avoid this herb. One should always consult their physician first or take herbal remedies only under a doctor's direction or when clinically proven safe for a particular condition.

Drug / Herbal Interaction

Drug reactions with other antiplatelets including Plavix® and Ticlid® are reason for concern. Also caution should be taken with use of heparin and warfarin. There is also a cautionary warning with use while taking long term Aspirin® (ASA) for its anti-clotting activity.

Because it can enhance the immune system, concomitant use with immunosupressants in transplant patients is cautioned. Jiaogulan can reverse the effects of Imuran, CellCept, cyclosporine, Rapamune and Zenapak.

There are a few herbal interactions that can occur. The herbs Danshen, Devil's Claw, Eleuthero, Garlic, Ginger, Ginkgo, Horse Chestnut, Panax Ginseng, and Papain should be taken with caution as they can increase the bleeding-time when used in conjunction with Jiaogulan.

Appendix

Table 1

List of other Primary Adaptogens:

Panax Ginseng
Ashwaganda (Withania somnifera)
Schizandra (*Schizandra chinensis*) Chinese magnolia berries
Reishi (Ganoderma lucidum)
Astragalus (Astragalus membranaceous)
Licorice (Glycyrrhiza glabra)
Cordyceps (cordyceps sinensis)
Gotu Kola

Other Secondary Adaptogen Herbs:

Wild Oats (Avena sativa)
Fo-ti or Ho Shou Wu (Polygonum multiflorum)
Burdock (Arctium lappa)
Suma (Pfaffia paniculata)
Tinospora cordifolia
Picrorrhiza kurroa
Momordica charantia
Terminalia chebula
Piper longum
Emblica officinalis
Centella asiatica
Leuzea carthamoides (Russian Leuzea)

Bacopa (bacopa monnieri)
Holy Basil (ocimum sanctum)
Chickpea (Cer arietinum)
Maca (Lepidium peruvianum Chacon, Lepidium meyenii)
Ligustrum (Ligustrum lucidum)
Andrographis paniculata (Acanthaceae)
Arogyappcha (Trichopus zeylanicus)
Guarana

Table 2

Diagram of the
Hypothalamus-Pituitary-Adrenal Axis

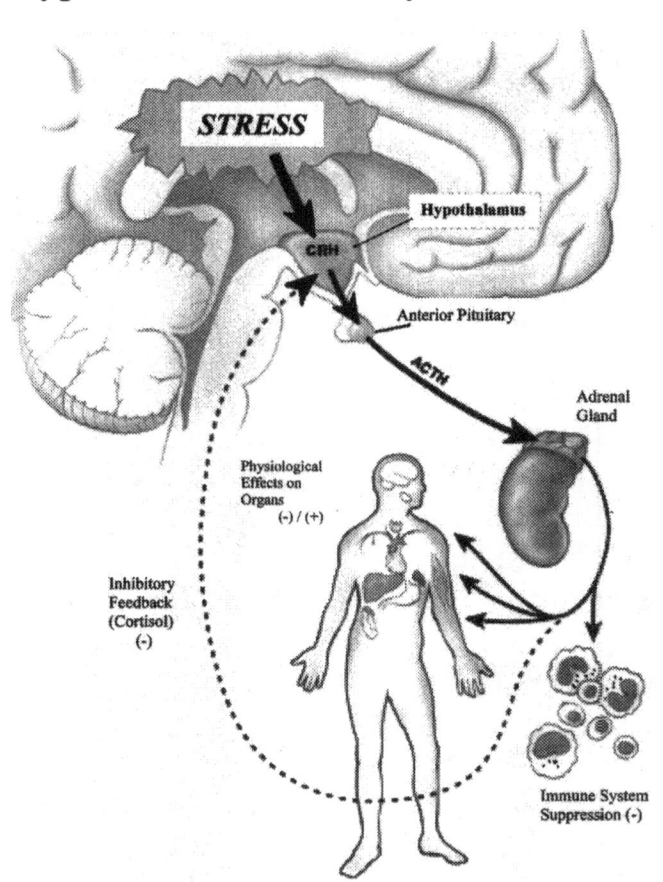

CRF—corticotropin-releasing factor
ACTH—adrenocorticotropic hormone

Stress induced release of CRF with a rise in ACTH causing Cortisol release from the Adrenal Glands. This has a negative effect on the Immune System and other organs of the body. Cortisol gives negative feedback to the hypothalamus thus reducing CRF levels.

Table 3

Buyers Guide

This list is intended to assist the reader in obtaining quality, standardized herbs.

Jagulana Herbal Products
PO Box 45
Badger, CA 93603-0045
(888) 465-3686
(559) 337-2188 www.immortalityherb.com
(Jiaogulan)

Oregon's Wild Harvest
PO Box 278
Sandy, OR 97055
(800) 316-6869
(503) 668-7713 www.oregonswildharvest.com
(Eleuthero)

Paradise Herbs, Inc.
8884 Warner Avenue, #153
Fountain Valley, CA 92708

(800) 691-2573
(714) 842-6355 www.paradiseherbs.com
(Rhodiola rosea, Eleuthero, Jiaogulan)

Planetary Formulas
PO Box 533
Soquel, CA 95073
(800) 606-6226
(831) 438-1700 www.planetaryformulas.com
(Rhodiola rosea)

PreGame Formulas
Sports Specific Nutrition, Inc
3665 River Trace Dr.
Alpharetta, GA 30022
(770) 619-4320 www.ssninc.net
(A formulation by Dr. Saleeby that includes
R. rosea and Eleuthero)

The Immortalitea Company
780 Knight Lane
El Dorado Hills, CA 95762
(530) 554-1389 www.immortalitea.com
(Jiaogulan)

Amber Keefer's Biography

Amber P. Keefer is a freelance writer who has had numerous articles published in: The Walking Magazine, Long-Term Care Interface, BBW Magazine, Chicago Parent Magazine, Chicago Baby Magazine, Metro Parent Magazine, Metro Baby Magazine, Family Digest Baby Magazine, All About Kids, Indy's Child, Home Education Magazine, Pittsburgh Parent, Atlanta Parent Magazine, South Florida

Parenting, San Diego Parent Magazine, Long Island Woman, Western New York Family Magazine, Parent Teen Magazine, Youth Magazine, Today's Family Matters, The Lutheran, Woman's Touch, Strawberry Saxifrage, The Messenger, Vermont Parent & Child Magazine, Big Apple Parent, Complementary Medicine News & others. She is a regular contributor to several columns in Family Digest Magazine and does PR writing and a monthly newsletter for a Continuing Care Community in the Montour County Area.

A lifelong resident of rural Central Pennsylvania, with a B.A. in Sociology and Criminal Justice from Bloomsburg University of Pennsylvania, Ms. Keefer writes about a wide range of topics, specializing in covering issues relating to education and health, particularly women's and children's health, including today's varying healthcare plans, safety and prevention, vision and dental care, chronic illness, stress-management, self-esteem and physical, social and emotional well-being for the entire family.

A former college administrator, Ms. Keefer has also previously worked in the Pennsylvania juvenile justice system. She is currently pursuing a Masters degree. She aided Dr. Saleeby as a co-author in writing selected chapters in this book.

Yusuf (J.P.) Saleeby, MD's Biography

Dr. Saleeby is a 1991 graduate from the Medical College of Georgia in Augusta, Georgia. Upon completion of post-graduate training at East Carolina University School of Medicine in Greenville, North Carolina, he relocated to Savannah, Georgia to practice emergency medicine. Since 2000 he has co-directed the Emergency Department at Liberty Regional Medical Center, Hinesville, GA and staffs the emergency room fulltime.

In addition to Emergency Medicine, he has also staffs the Juliet Gordon Low Federal Building's Federal Occupational Health center as chief medical officer. Dr. Saleeby received education in longevity and integrative medicine through association and membership at one time with the American Academy of Anti-Aging Medicine (A4M) and the American College for the Advancement of Medicine (ACAM). Most of his knowledge of adaptogen herbs comes from self-study in this area of medicine.

Dr. Saleeby founded the Saleeby Longevity Institute in Savannah, GA, which served the southeastern region from September 2000 until March 2004. In addition to his full time commitment to the emergency room he now practices longevity medicine with a focus on prevention and nutrition via telemedicine consultations (www.saleeby.net). Dr. Saleeby founded Vita Sanus Nurtracuticals (VSN) (www.vitasanus.com) in 1998 where he was able to formulate a line of pharmaceutical grade dietary supplements for his patients. He was commissioned by SSN, Inc to formulate a sports supplement (PreGame Golf & Tennis products) representing a number of adaptogen herbs that went to market in 2004.

Dr. Saleeby also holds post as an adjunct professor in the Graduate School of Nursing at Georgia Southern University, Statesboro, Georgia. He is a regional speaker on topics of integrative and preventive medicine and has been published in regional and national journals and magazines. He was past senior editor of the quarterly newsletter Complementary Medicine News, an integrative medicine newsletter. Most recently he has published articles related to health and wellness in local Georgia & South Carolina publications such as: Savannah Out Front, Coastal Health and Fitness Magazine, CARE Magazine, Connect Savannah. He has also been published in MountainX magazine, Asheville,

NC, Enigma Magazine, Chattanooga, TN, JIVE magazine, Atlanta, GA, DEEP Magazine, Southeastern USA.

The national journal American Fitness has recently published a number of his articles. He has been quoted in the New York Times, American Fitness Magazine, Medical Economics, Cortlandt Forum, and on regional TV and radio stations. He published his first e-book in 2002 and has been working on this book since 2003. Dr. Saleeby maintains a blog of his most current medical writings at www.docsaleeby.blogspot.com.

An avid oneophile he had co-founded a wine club in Savannah. Dr. Saleeby recently participated in Olympic style Weightifting with Team Savannah, and has attained top place finishes in his 94 kg Masters group at the Georgia Games and the Team Savannah Open competition in 2002 & 2003 and took the Silver Medal in the 2004 Senior National competition. He adores his two children Michael and Madison, enjoys world travel along with teaching others in the field of integrative medicine.

References

Introduction:

Lipnick RL, Filov VA., Nikolai Vasilyevich Lazarev, toxicologist and pharmacologist, comes in from the cold. Trends Pharmacol Sci. 1992 Feb;13(2):56-60.

Dietary Supplement Health and Education Act of 1994, Public Law 103-417, 103rd Congress (1994), http://www. fda.gov/opacom/laws/dshea.html (December 22, 2005)

Rhodiola rosea:

Kelly, GS, Rhodiola rosea: A Possible Plant Adaptogen, Alternative Medicine Review, Thorne Research, 2001;6(3):293-302

Waggoner, B.W., Linneaus (2000), http://www.ucmp. berkeley.edu/history/linnaeus.html (December 22, 2005)

Petkov VD, Yonkov D, Mosharoff A, et al. Effects of alcohol aqueous extract from Rhodiola rosea L. roots on learning and memory. Acta Physiol Pharmacol Bulg 1986;12:3-16.

Brekhman II, Dardymov IV. New substances of plant origin which increase nonspecific resistance. Ann Rev Pharmacol 1969;9:419-430.

Lishmanov IB, Trifonova ZV, Tsibin AN, et al. Plasma beta-endorphin and stress hormones in stress and adaptation. Biull Eksp Biol Med 1987;103:422-424. [Article in Russian]

Linh PT, Kim YH, Hong SP, et al. Quantitative determination of salidroside and tyrosol from the underground part of Rhodiola rosea by high performance liquid chromatography. Arch Pharm Res 2000;23:349-352.

Lee MW, Lee YA, Park HM, et al. Antioxidative phenolic compounds from the roots of Rhodiola sachalinensis. A. Bor. Arch Pharm Res 2000;23:455-458.

Ohsugi M, Fan W, Hase K, et al. Active-oxygen scavenging activity of traditional nourishing-tonic herbal medicines and active constituents of Rhodiola sacra. J Ethnopharmacol 1999;67:111-119.

Visioli F, Galli C, Bornet F, et al. Olive oil phenolics are dose-dependently absorbed in humans. FEBS Lett 2000;468:159-160.

Bonanome A, Pagnan A, Caruso D, et al. Evidence of postprandial absorption of olive oil phenols in humans. Nutr Metab Cardiovasc Dis 2000;10:111-120.

de la Puerta R, Ruiz Gutierrez V, Hoult JR. Inhibition of leukocyte 5-lipoxygenase by phenolics from virgin olive oil. Biochem Pharmacol 1999;57:445-449.

Boon-Niermeijer EK, van den Berg A, Wikman G, Wiegant FA. Phyto-adaptogens protect against environmental stress-induced death of embryos from the freshwater snail Lymnaea stagnalis. Phytomedicine 2000;7:389-399.

Stancheva SL, Mosharrof A. Effect of the extract of Rhodiola rosea L. on the content of the brain biogenic monamines. Med Physiol 1987;40:85-87.

Maslova LV, Kondrat'ev BI, Maslov LN, Lishmanov IB. The cardioprotective and antiadrenergic activity of an extract of Rhodiola rosea in stress. Eksp Klin Farmakol 1994;57:61-63.

Lishmanov IB, Maslova LV, Maslov LN, Dan'shina EN. The anti-arrhythmia effect of Rhodiola rosea and its possible mechanism. Biull Eksp Biol Med 1993;116:175-176.

Maimeskulova LA, Maslov LN, Lishmanov IB, Krasnov EA. The participation of the mu-, delta- and kappa-opioid receptors in the realization of the anti-arrhythmia effect of Rhodiola rosea. Eksp Klin Farmakol 1997;60:38-39.

Lishmanov IB, Naumova AV, Afanas'ev SA, Maslov LN. Contribution of the opioid system to realization of inotropic effects of Rhodiola rosea extracts in ischemic and reperfusion heart damage in vitro. Eksp Klin Farmakol 1997;60:34-36.

Azizov AP, Seifulla RD. The effect of elton, leveton, fitoton and adapton on the work capacity of experimental animals. Eksp Klin Farmakol 1998;61:61-63.

Lazarova MB, Petkov VD, Markovska VL, et al. Effects of meclofenoxate and Extr. Rhodiolae roseae L. on electroconvulsive shock-impaired learning and memory in rats. Methods Find Exp Clin Pharmacol 1986;8:547-552.

Afanas'ev SA, Alekseeva ED, Bardamova IB, et al. Cardiac contractile function following acute cooling of the body and the adaptogenic correction of its disorders. Biull Eksp Biol Med 1993;116:480-483.

Maimeskulova LA, Maslov LN. The anti-arrhythmia action of an extract of Rhodiola rosea and of n-tyrosol in models of experimental arrhythmias. Eksp Klin Farmakol 1998;61:37-40.

Udintsev SN, Shakhov VP. The role of humoral factors of regenerating liver in the development of experimental tumors and the effect of Rhodiola rosea extract on this process. Neoplasma 1991;38:323-331.

Udintsev SN, Schakhov VP. Decrease of cyclophosphamide haematotoxicity by Rhodiola rosea root extract in mice with Ehrlich and Lewis transplantable tumors. Eur J Cancer 1991;27:1182.

Udintsev SN, Krylova SG, Fomina TI. The enhancement of the efficacy of adriamycin by using hepatoprotectors of plant origin in metastases of Ehrlich's adenocarcinoma to the liver in mice. Vopr Onkol 1992;38:1217-1222.

Germano C, Ramazanov Z, Bernal Suarez M. Arctic Root (Rhodiola Rosea): The Powerful New Ginseng Alternative. New York, NY: Kensington Publishing Corp; 1999.

Darbinyan V, Kteyan A, Panossian A, et al. Rhodiola rosea in stress induced fatigue a double blind cross-over study of a standardized extract SHR-5 with a repeated low-dose regimen on the mental performance of healthy physicians during night duty. Phytomedicine 2000;7:365-371.

Spasov AA, Wikman GK, Mandrikov VB, et al. A double-blind, placebo-controlled pilot study of the stimulating and adaptogenic effect of Rhodiola rosea SHR-5 extract on the fatigue of students caused by stress during an examination period with a repeated low-dose regimen. Phytomedicine 2000;7:85-89.

Baranov AI. Medicinal uses of ginseng and related plants in the Soviet Union: recent trends in the Soviet literature. J Ethnopharmacol 1982;6:339-353.

Hiai S, Yokoyama H, Oura H, Yano S. Stimulation of pituitary-adrenocortical system by ginseng saponin. Endocrinol Jpn 1979;26:661-665.

Fulder SJ. Ginseng and the hypothalamic-pituitary control of stress. Am J Chin Med 1981;9:112-118.

Golotin VG, Gonenko VA, Zimina VV, et al. Effect of ionol and eleutherococcus on changes of the hypophyseo-adrenal system in rats under extreme conditions. Vopr Med Khim 1989;35:35-37.

Ramazanov, Z. et al. New secrets of effective natural stress and weight management, using Rhodiola rosea and Rhodendron caucasicum. ATN/Safe Goods Publishing, (1999) CT.

Duhan, O.M. et al. The antimutagenic activity of biomass extracts from the cultured cells of medicinal plants in the Ames test. Tsitol Genet Nov-Dec (1999) 33(6): 19-25

Bocharova OA et.al. The effect of a Rhodiola rosea extract on the incidence of recurrences of a superficial bladder cancer (experimental clinical research). Urol Nefrol (Mosk) Mar-Apr (1995) (2): 46-7

Salikhova RA et.al, Effect of Rhodiola rosea on the yield of mutation alteration and DNA repair in bone marrow cells. Patol Fiziol Exsp Ter Oct-Dec. (1997) (4): 22-4

Eleuthero:

RxList.com: Siberian Ginseng (Eleutherococcus senticosus) http://www.rxlist.com/cgi/alt/ginseng_sib_faq.htm, last updated 12-8-2004 (December 22, 2005)

Canada's Digital Collections, Hans Selye: Understanding Stress, http://www.collections.gc.ca/heirloom_series/volume4/222-223.htm (December 22, 2005)

Blumenthal M, ed. The Complete German Commission E Monographs. Boston, Mass: Integrative Medicine Communications; 1998:124-125.

Bucci LR. Selected herbals and human exercise performance. Am J Clin Nutr. 2000;72(suppl):624S-636S.

Fugh-Berman A. Herb-drug interactions. Lancet. 2000;355:134-138.

Glatthaar-Saalmuller B, Sacher F, Esperester A. Antiviral activity of an extract derived from roots of Eleutherococcus senticosus. Antiviral Res. 2001;50(3):223-8.

Gyllenhaal C, Merritt SL, Peterson SD, Block KI, Gochenour T. Efficacy and safety of herbal stimulants and sedatives in sleep disorders. Sleep Med Rev. 2000;4(2):229-251.

Harkey MR, Henderson GL, Gershwin ME, Stern JS, Hackman RM. Variability in commercial ginseng products: an analysis of 25 preparations. Am J Clin Nutr. 2001;73:1101-1106.

Kelly GS. Nutritional and botanical interventions to assist with the adaptation to stress. Alt Med Rev. 1999;4(4):249-265.

Koren G, Randor S, Martin S, Danneman D. Maternal ginseng use associated with neonatal androgenization [letter]. JAMA. 1990;264(22):2866.

McRae S. Elevated serum digoxin levels in a patient taking digoxin and Siberian ginseng. Can Med Assoc J. 1996;155:293-295.

Miller LG. Herbal medicinals: selected clinical considerations focusing on known or potential drug-herb interactions. Arch Intern Med. 1998;158(20):2200-2211.

Newall CA, Anderson LA, Phillipson JD. Herbal Medicines: A Guide for Health Care Professionals. London, England: The Pharmaceutical Press; 1996:141-144.

Ott BR, Owens NJ. Complementary and alternative medicines for Alzheimer's disease. J Geriatr Psychiatry Neurol. 1998;11:163-173.

Pizzorno JE, Murray MT, eds. Textbook of Natural Medicine. New York, NY: Churchill-Livingstone; 1999:433-434;531-532;713-717;1385-1386.

Sinclair S. Male infertility: nutritional and environmental considerations. Alt Med Rev. 2000;5(1):28-38.

Vogler BK, Pittler MH, Ernst E. The efficacy of ginseng. A systematic review of randomized clinical trials. Eur J Clin Pharmacol. 1999;55:567-575.

White L, Mavor S. Kids, Herbs, Health. Loveland, Colo: Interweave Press; 1998:22, 40.

Williams M. Immuno-protection against herpes simplex type II infection by eleutherococcus root extract. Int J Alt Comp Med. 1995;13:9-12.

Winther K, Ranlov C, Rein E, Mehlsen J. Russian root (Siberian ginseng) improves cognitive functions in middle-aged people, whereas Ginkgo biloba seems effective only in the elderly. J Neurol Sci. 1997;150:S90.

Wong AHC, Smith M, Boon HS. Herbal remedies in psychiatric practice. Arch Gen Psychiatry. 1998;55:1033-1044.

Asano K, Takahashi T, Miyashita M, et al. Effect of Eleutherococcus senticosus extract on human physical working capacity. Planta Medica. 1986;(3):175-177.

Awang DV. Siberian ginseng toxicity may be case of mistaken identity. Canadian Medical Association Journal. 1996;155(9):1237.

Awang DV. What in the name of Panax are those other "ginsengs"? HerbalGram. 2003;57:35-40.

Baranov AI. Medicinal uses of ginseng and related plants in the Soviet Union: recent trends in the Soviet literature. Journal of Ethnopharmacology. 1982;6(3):339-353.

Bazaz'ian GG, Liapina LA, Pastorova VE, Zvereva EG. Effect of Eleutherococcus on the functional status of the anticoagulation system in older animals. Fiziol Zh SSSR Im I M Sechenova. 1987;73(10):1390-1395.

Blumenthal M., Farm Bill bans use of name "ginseng" on non-Panax species: "Siberian ginseng" no longer allowed as commercial term [press release]. Austin, Texas: American Botanical Council; Fall 2002.

Cicero AF, Derosa G, Brillante R, Bernardi R, Nascetti S, Gaddi A. Effects of Siberian ginseng (Eleutherococcus senticosus maxim.) on elderly quality of life: a randomized clinical trial. Archives of Gerontology and Geriatrics Supplement. 2004;(9):69-73.

Dasgupta A, Wu S, Actor J, Olsen M, Wells A, Datta P. Effect of Asian and Siberian ginseng on serum digoxin measurement by five digoxin immunoassays. Significant variation in digoxin-like immunoreactivity among commercial ginsengs. American Journal of Clinical Pathology. 2003;119(2):298-303.

Davydov M, Krikorian AD. Eleutherococcus senticosus (Rupr. & Maxim.) Maxim. (Araliaceae) as an adaptogen: a closer look. Journal of Ethnopharmacology. 2000;72(3):345-393.

Deyama T, Nishibe S, Nakazawa Y. Constituents and pharmacological effects of Eucommia and Siberian ginseng. Acta Pharmacol Sin. 2001;22(12):1057-1070.

Donovan JL, DeVane CL, Chavin KD, Taylor RM, Markowitz JS. Siberian ginseng (Eleutheroccus [sic] senticosus) effects on CYP2D6 and CYP3A4 activity in normal volunteers. Drug Metabolism and Disposition. 2003;31(5):519-522.

Dowling EA, Redondo DR, Branch JD, Jones S, McNabb G, Williams MH. Effect of Eleutherococcus senticosus on submaximal and maximal exercise performance. Medical Science in Sports and Exercise. 1996;28:482-489.

Drozd J, Sawicka T, Prosinska J. Estimation of humoral activity of Eleutherococcus senticosus. Acta Pol Pharm. 2002;59(5):395-401.

Eschbach LF, Webster MJ, Boyd JC, McArthur PD, Evetovich TK. The effect of Siberian ginseng (Eleutherococcus senticosus) on substrate utilization and performance. International Journal of Sports Nutrition and Exercise Metabolism. 2000;10(4):444-451.

Gaffney BT, Hugel HM, Rich PA. The effects of Eleutherococcus senticosus and Panax ginseng on steroidal hormone indices of stress and lymphocyte subset numbers in endurance athletes. Life Sciences. 2001;70(4):431-442.

Gaffney BT, Hugel HM, Rich PA. Panax ginseng and Eleutherococcus senticosus may exaggerate an already existing biphasic response to stress via inhibition of enzymes which limit the binding of stress hormones to their receptors. Medical Hypotheses. 2001;56(5):567-572.

Glatthaar-Saalmuller B, Sacher F, Esperester A. Antiviral activity of an extract derived from roots of Eleutherococcus senticosus. Antiviral Research. 2001;50(3):223-228.

Hacker B, Medon PJ. Cytotoxic effects of Eleutherococcus senticosus aqueous extracts in combination with N6-(delta 2-isopentenyl)-adenosine and 1-beta-D-arabinofuranosylcytosine against L1210 leukemia cells. Journal of Pharmaceutical Science. 1984;73(2):270-272.

Harkey MR, Henderson GL, Zhou L, et al. Effects of Siberian ginseng (Eleutherococcus senticosus) on c-DNA-expressed P450 drug metabolizing enzymes. Alternative Therapy. 2001;7:S14.

Hartz AJ, Bentler S, Noyes R, et al. Randomized controlled trial of Siberian ginseng for chronic fatigue. Psychological Medicine. 2004;34(1):51-61.

HealthNotes, Inc. Eleuthero. 2002. http://www.mycustompak.com/healthNotes/Herb/Eleuthero.htm Accessed March 28, 2003 by another author. (not found December 22, 2005)

Henderson GL, Harkey MR, Gershwin ME, Hackman RM, Stern JS, Stresser DM Effects of ginseng components on c-DNA-expressed cytochrome P450 enzyme catalytic activity. Life Sciences. 1999;65(15):PL209-PL214.

Hikino H, Takahashi M, Otake K, Konno C. Isolation and hypoglycemic activity of eleutherans A, B, C, D, E, F, and G: glycans of Eleutherococcus senticosus roots. Journal of Natural Products. 1986;49(2):293-297.

Jellin JM, Gregory P, Batz F, Hitchens K, et al, eds. Pharmacist's Letter/Prescriber's Letter. Natural Medicines Comprehensive Database, 3rd Edition. Stockton CA: Therapeutic Research Facility, 2000.

Jeong HJ, Koo HN, Myung NI, et al. Inhibitory effects of mast cell-mediated allergic reactions by cell cultured Siberian Ginseng. Immunopharmacology and Immunotoxicology. 2001;23(1):107-117.

Kwan CY, Zhang WB, Sim SM, Deyama T, Nishibe S. Vascular effects of Siberian ginseng (Eleutherococcus senticosus): endothelium-dependent NO- and EDHF-mediated relaxation depending on vessel size. Naunyn Schmiedebergs Arch Pharmacol. 2004;369(5):473-480.

Lewis WH, Zenger VE, Lynch RG. No adaptogen response of mice to ginseng and Eleutherococcus infusions. Journal of Ethnopharmacology. 1983;8(2):209-214.

McRae S. Elevated serum digoxin levels in a patient taking digoxin and Siberian ginseng. Canadian Medical Association Journal. 1996;155(3):293-295.

Medon PJ, Ferguson PW, Watson CF. Effects of Eleutherococcus senticosus extracts on hexobarbital metabolism in vivo and in vitro. Journal of Ethnopharmacology. 1984;10(2):235-241.

Park EJ, Nan JX, Zhao YZ, et al. Water-soluble polysaccharide from Eleutherococcus senticosus stems attenuates fulminant hepatic failure induced by D-galactosamine and lipopolysaccharide in mice. Basic Clinical Pharmacology and Toxicology. 2004;94(6):298-304.

Rogala E, Skopinska-Rozewska E, Sawicka T, Sommer E, Prosinska J, Drozd J. The influence of Eleuterococcus [sic] senticosus on cellular and humoral immunological response of mice. Polish Journal of Veterinary Science. 2003;6(Suppl 3):37-39.

Scholz MW, Sacher F, Aicher B. The synthesis of RANTES, G-CSF, IL-4, IL-5, IL-6, IL-12, and IL-13 in human whole blood cultures is modulated by an extract from Eleutherococcus senticosus L. roots. Phytotherapy Research. 2001;15:268-270.

Shi Z, Liu C, Li R. Effect of a mixture of Acanthopanax senticosus and Elsholtzia splendens on serum-lipids in patients with hyperlipemia. Zhong Xi Yi Jie He Za Zhi. 1990;10(3):132 and 155-156.

Sievenpiper JL, Arnason JT, Leiter LA, Vuksan V. Decreasing, null and increasing effects of eight popular types of ginseng on acute postprandial glycemic indices in healthy humans: the role of ginsenosides. Journal of the American College of Nutrition. 2004;23(3):248-258.

Szolomicki S, Samochowiec L, Wojcicki J, Drozdzik M. The influence of active components of Eleutherococcus senticosus on cellular defense and physical fitness in man. Phytotherapy Research. 2000;14(3):30-35.

Tutel'yan AV, Klebanov GI, Il'ina SE, Lyubitskii OB. Comparative study of antioxidant properties of immunoregulatory peptides. Bulletin of Experimental Biology in Medicine. 2003;136(2):155-158.

Wang H, Actor JK, Indrigo J, Olsen M, Dasgupta A. Asian and Siberian ginseng as a potential modulator of immune function: an in vitro cytokine study using mouse macrophages. Clinica Chimica Acta. 2003;327(1-2):123-128.

Webb D. Eleuthero—a detailed review of its reputed effect as an adaptogen. HerbalGram. February 6, 2001.

Yi JM, Hong SH, Kim JH, Kim HK, Song HJ, Kim HM. Effect of Acanthopanax senticosus stem on mast cell-dependent anaphylaxis. Journal of Ethnopharmacology. 2002;79(3):347-352.

Zand J. Siberian ginseng. The herb for energy and stress. Health World Online. http://healthy.net/asp/templates/article. asp?PageType=Article& ID=917. Accessed May 23, 2003 by another author. (not present on December 22, 2005)

Awang, D.V.C. Maternal Use of Ginseng and Neonatal Androgenization. JAMA, April 10, 1991; 265(14):1828.

Awang, D.V.C. Maternal Use of Ginseng and Neonatal Androgenization. JAMA, July 17, 1991;266(3):363.

Blumenthal, M., T. Hall, R. Rister, B Steinhoff (eds.), S. Klein, R. Rister (trans.). The German Commission E Monographs. Austin, Texas: American Botanical Council. 1996.

Baranov, A.I. On a Technical English Name for Eleutherococcus. Taxon 1979; 28:586-587.

Duke, J. A. and E.S. Ayensu. Medicinal Plants of China. 2 vols. Algonac, MI: Reference Publications. 1985.

Farnsworth, N.R., A. D. Kinghorn, D.D. Soejarto and D. P. Waller. Siberian Ginseng (Eleutherococcus senticosus):

Current Status as an Adaptogen. pp. 155-215. In H. Wagner, H.Hikino and N.R. Farnsworth (eds.). Economic and Medicinal Plant Research. Vol. 1. Orlando, FL: Academic Press. 1985

Foster, S. and C. X. Yue. Herbal Emmissaries: Bringing Chinese Herbs to the West. Rochester, Vt: Healing Arts Press. 1992.

Fulder, S. The Drug That Builds Russians, New Sci. 1980;21:576-579.

Halstead, BW. and L.L. Hood. Eleutherococcus senticosus Siberian Ginseng: An Introduction to the Concept of Adaptogenic Medicine. Long Beach, CA: Oriental Healing Arts Institute. 1984.

Hu, S.Y. (letter to S. Foster) p. 44 In S. Foster. Ginseng: Are You Confused: A Look at Controversy in the Herb World. Well-Being No. 46: 43-50 (October, 1979).

Hu, S.Y. Eleutherococcus vs. Acanthopanax. Journ. Arn. Arb. 1980; 61: 107-111.

Hu, S.Y. An Enumeration of Chinese Materia Medica. Hong Kong: The Chinese University Press. 1980.

Lucas R. Eleuthero (Siberian Ginseng) Health Herb of Russia. Spokane WA: R&M Books. 1973.

McCaleb, R. Dr. I.I. Brekhman (interview) HerbalGram 1988;16:11-12.

Ohwi, J. Flora of Japan. Washington, D.C.: Smithsonian Institution. 1965.

Pharmacopeia Committee of the Ministry of Health. Pharmacopeia of the People's Republic of China (Zhong Hua Ren Min Gong He Guo Yao, Dian, Ti Bu). Part 1. Beijing: People's Health Publishing House and Chemical Industry Publishing House. 1985.

Poyarkova, A.I. Eleutherococcus pp. 16-23. In B.K. Shishkin. Flora of the U.S.S.R. (1950) Translated from Russian. Jerusalem: Israel Program for Scientific Translations. 1973.

Soejarto, D.D. and N. R. Farnsworth. The Correct Name for Siberian Ginseng. Bot. Mus. Leafl., Harv. Univ. 1978;26 (9-10): 339-341.

Wagner, H. and A. Proksch. Immunostimulatory Drugs of Fungi and Higher Plants. pp. 111-153. In H. Wagner, H. Hikino and N.R. Farnsworth (eds.). Economic and Medicinal Plant Research. Vol. 1. Orlando, FL: Academic Press. 1985.

Waller, D. P., A. M. Martin, N. R. Farnsworth, and D.V.C. Awang. Lack of Androgenicity of Siberian ginseng. JAMA, May 6, 1992; 267(17):2329.

Yueh, C.H. 1987. Personal communication. In report by Steven Foster on www.herbalgram.org on Eleutherococcus senticosus, 1990 American Botanical Council, Revised edition 1996 American Botanical Council.

Jiaogulan:

Cheng, J.G., et al. Investigation of the plant jiaogulan and its analogous herb, Wulianmei. Zhong Cao Yao. Chinese. 1990. 21(9): 424.

Li Shi-Zhen (Ming dynasty): Ben Chao Gangu Mu (Compendium of Materia Medica) Vol. 2. People's Health Publisher. Chinese. 1985. p. 1326.

Wu, Qi-Jun. (Qing dynasty). Zi Wu Ming Shi Tu Kau (Textual Investigation of Herbal Plants) Vol. 2, Shang Wu Publishing House. Chinese. 1957. p. 559.

Qu, Jing and combined research group of Traditional Chinese/Western Medicine, Yunnan. Study of the therapeutic effects of Chinese herb, jiaogulan in 537 cases of chronic tracheo-bronchitis. Zhong Chao Yao Tong Xun (Bulletin of Chinese Herbs and Medicines). Chinese. 1972. (2): 24.

Wu, Y.G., et al. (ed), Dictionary of Chinese Materia Medica Vol2, p.1088, Shanghai Science and Technological Publishing House, Shanghai, 1st. ed. Chinese. 1998.

Nagai, Masahiro, et al. Two Glycosides of a Novel Dammarane Alcohol from Gynostemma pentaphyllum. Chem. Pharm. Bull. 1981. 29(3): 779-83.

Izawa, Kazuo. Color Encyclopedia of Medicinal Herbs. Jpn. 1998: 458.

Nagai, Masahiro, et al. Abstracts of Papers. The 23rd Meeting of the Japanese Society of Pharmacognosy. Jpn. Nov. 1976: 37.

Takemoto, Tsunematsu, et al. Health Before You Know It.- Amachazuru. Eng. Yutaka Nakano Shobo 1984.

Takemoto, Tsunematsu, et al. Studies of the constituents of Gynostemma pentaphyllum Makino. I. Structures of

Gypenosides I-XIV. Yakugakuzasshi. Jpn. 1983. 103(2): 173-185.

Bergner, Paul. The Healing Power of Ginseng. Prima Publishing. 1996. 107.

Yoshikawa, K., et al. Studies on the constituents of Cucurbitaceae plants. XVIII. On the Saponin constituents of Gynostemma pentaphyllum Makino (13) Yakugaku Zasshi. Jpn. 1987. 107: 361-366.

Arichi, Shigeru, et al. Saponins of Gynostemma pentaphyllum as tonics. Kokai Tokkyo Koho. Jpn. 1985. 60(105): 626.

Arichi, Shigeru, et al. Saponins of Gynostemma pentaphyllum as neoplasm inhibitors. Kokai Tokkyo Koho. Jpn. 1985. 60(105): 627.

Arichi, Shigeru, et al. Prevention of glucocorticoid side effects by saponins of Gynostemma pentaphyllum. Kokai Tokkyo Koho. Jpn. 1985. 60(105): 625.

Guangxi Ribao (Guangxi Daily Newspaper). Chinese. March 4, 1972.

Wu, Y.G., et al. (ed), Dictionary of Chinese materia Medica Vol 2, p. 1088. Chinese. Shanghai Science and Technological Publishing House, Shanghai, 1st. ed. 1998.

Health Sciences Institute Members Alert for July 2000

Asia Pacific Journal of Pharmacology, 5(4):321-322, 1990

Journal of Guiyang Medical College, 18(4):261, 1993

Journal of Guiyang Medical College, 18(3):146, 1993

Cancer Biotherapy, 8(3):263, 1993

Journal of West China University of Medical Sciences, 26(4):430-432, 1995

Zhong Yao Li Yu Lin Chuang, 7(2):39, 1991

Guizhou Medical Journal, 20(1), 1996

Zhongguo Yaolixue Zazhi, 4(1):17-20, 1990

Journal of Pharmacology, 5(4):321-322, 1990

Industiral Hygiene and Professional Disease, 24(2):74, 1998

Hunan Journal of Traditional Chinese Medicine, 9(4):11, 1993

Research on Chinese Herbs, 4:136, 1996

Klotter, J., Townsend Letter for Doctors and Patients, Feb-March, 2004

Aktan F, Henness S, Roufogalis BD, Ammit AJ. Gypenosides derived from Gynostemma pentaphyllum suppress NO synthesis in murine macrophages by inhibiting iNOS enzymatic activity and attenuating NF-kappaB-mediated iNOS protein expression. Nitric Oxide. 2003;8(4):235-242.

Anon. Fibrosis. In: Beers, MH, Berkow R, Burs M (eds). The Merck Manual of Diagnosis and Therapy, 17th ed. Whitehouse Station, New Jersey: Merck & Co, Inc; 1999.

Blumert M, Liu JL (Eds). Jiaogulan (Gynostemma pentaphyllum)—China's "Immortality" Herb. Badger, California: Torchlight Publishing; 1999.

Chan LY, Chiu PY, Lau TK. An in-vitro study of ginsenoside Rb(1)-induced teratogenicity using a whole rat embryo culture model. Human Reproduction. 2003;18(10):2166-2168.

Chen JC, Chung JG, Chen LD. Gypenoside induces apoptosis in human Hep3B and HA22T tumour cells. Cytobios. 1999;100(393):37-48.

Chen JC, Tsai CC, Chen LD, Chen HH, Wang WC. Therapeutic effect of gypenoside on chronic liver injury and fibrosis induced by CCl4 in rats. American Journal of Chinese Medicine. 2000;28(2):175-185.

Cui J, Eneroth P, Bruhn JG. Gynostemma pentaphyllum: identification of major sapogenins and differentiation from Panax species. European Journal of Pharmaceutical Sciences. 1999;8(3):187-191.

Francis G, Kerem Z, Makkar HP, Becker K. The biological action of saponins in animal systems: a review. British Journal of Nutrition. 2002;88(6):587-605.

Jellin JM, Gregory P, Batz F, Hitchens K, et al, eds. Pharmacist's Letter/Prescriber's Letter. Natural Medicines Comprehensive Database, 3rd Edition. Stockton CA: Therapeutic Research Facility, 2000.

la Cour B, Molgaard P, Yi Z. Traditional Chinese medicine in treatment of hyperlipidaemia. Journal of Ethnopharmacology. 1995;46(2):125-129.

Li L, Jiao L, Lau BH. Protective effect of gypenosides against oxidative stress in phagocytes, vascular endothelial cells and liver microsomes. Cancer Biotherapy. 1993;8(3):263-272.

Lin CC, Huang PC, Lin JM. Antioxidant and hepatoprotective effects of Anoectochilus formosanus and Gynostemma pentaphyllum. American Journal of Chinese Medicine. 2000;28(1):87-96.

Lin JM, Lin CC, Chiu HF, Yang JJ, Lee SG. Evaluation of the anti-inflammatory and liver-protective effects of anoectochilus formosanus, ganoderma lucidum and gynostemma pentaphyllum in rats. American Journal of Chinese Medicine. 1993;21(1):59-69.

Purmova J, Opletal L. Phytotherapeutic aspects of diseases of the cardiovascular system. 5. Saponins and possibilities of their use in prevention and therapy. Ceska Slov Farm. 1995;44(5):246-251.

Qi G, Zhang L, Li C. Influence of gypenoside on serum lipoprotein and atherosclerosis in hyperlipidaemia animals. Zhongguo Zhong Yao Za Zhi. 1996;21(9):562-564

Qi G, Zhang L, Xie WL, Chen XY, Li JS. Protective effect of gypenosides on DNA and RNA of rat neurons in cerebral ischemia-reperfusion injury. Acta Pharmacol Sin. 2000;21(12):1193-1196.

Tan H, Liu ZL, Liu MJ. Antithrombotic effect of Gynostemma pentaphyllum. Zhingguo Zhong Xi Yi Jie He Za Zhi 1993;13(5):278-280.

Tanner MA, Bu X, Steimle JA, Myers PR. The direct release of nitric oxide by gypenosides derived from the herb Gynostemma pentaphyllum. Nitric Oxide. 1999;3(5):359-365.

Wang C, Wang X, Li Y, Deng S, Jiang Y, Yue L. A preliminary observation of preventive and blocking effect of Gynostemma pentaphyllum (Thunb) Makino on esophageal cancer in rats. Hua Xi Yi Ke Da Xue Xue Bao. 1995;26(4):430-432.

Wang QF, Chen JC, Hsieh SJ, Cheng CC, Hsu SL. Regulation of Bcl-2 family molecules and activation of caspase cascade involved in gypenosides-induced apoptosis in human hepatoma cells. Cancer Letters. 2002;183(2):169-178.

Zhang C, Yang X, Xu L. Immunomodulatory action of the total saponin of Gynostemma pentaphylla. Zhong Xi Yi Jie He Za Zhi. 1990;10(2):96-70.

Zhou Z, Tang G, Zhong W. [Experimental study on the influence of Gynostemma pentaphyllam [sic] Mak upon point mutation of Ha-ras oncogene in blocking leukoplakia from canceration. Zhonghua Kou Qiang Yi Xue Za Zhi. 2000;35(2):91-94.

Zhou Z, Wang Y, Zhou Y. The effect of Gynostemma pentaphyllum mak (GP) on carcinogenesis of the golden hamster cheek pouch induced by DMBA. Zhonghua Kou Qiang Yi Xue Za Zhi. 1996;31(5):267-270.

Zhou Z, Wang Y, Zhou Y, Zhang S. Effect of gynostemma pentaphyllum mak on carcinomatous conversions of golden hamster cheek pouches induced by dimethylbenzanthracene:

a histological study. Chinese Medical Journal (English Edition). 1998;111(9):847-850.

Flora of China Study. Missouri Botanical Garden. www. mobot.org June 1998. (December 22, 2005)

Mount Fanjing Biosphere Reserve. World Network of Biosphere Reserves. Man and Biosphere Programme of UNESCO. 1986.

Zhu, SX et al. Detection of gypenoside concentration in jiaogulan harvested at different times. Hunan Zhongyi Zazhi. Chinese. 1990; 6(4): 52.

Xiao, XH et al. Distribution and resources of Genus Gynostemma in Shichuan. Zhong Yao Cai. Chinese. 1991; 14(3): 16.

Huang, TF. New techniques for heightening the production quantity of jiaogulan in cultivation. Zhong Cao Yao. Chinese. 1993; 24(12): 648.

Seong, JD et al. Characteristics, distribution and propagation methods of medicinal crop Dungkulcha, Gynostemma pentaphyllum. Res. Rep. Rural Dev. Adm (Suweon) 31(3 Upland Ind. Crops) Philippine. 1989; 57-61.

Shi Jianping, et al. Effects of Gynostemma Pentaphyllum on patients with hyperlipidemia. Journal of Norman Bethune University of Medical Science, 2001; vol.1, No.4, p343.

Lin Chuandi, et al. Safety and Efficacy of Gynostemma Pentaphyllum on regulating lipoprotein. Journal of Guangdong Medical College 2001 Vol.19 No.3 :.200-201.

Kang Jinian, et al. Effects of Gynostemma Pentaphyllum in Blood Lipid Metabolism. Chinese Traditional and Herbal Drugs 2000; 31 (10): 770-771.

Kimura, Y. et al. Effects of crude saponins of Gynostemma pentaphyllum on lipid metabolism. Shoyakugaku Zasshi. Japanese. 1983; 37(3): 272-275.

Yu, C. Therapeutic effect of a gypenosides tablet on 32 patients with hyperlipaemia. Journal of the integrated medicine of western and traditional Chinese medicines, HuBei State, China. 1993. 15(3): 21.

Wang Juntang, et al. Therapeutic observation of Gynostemma Pentaphyllum's effects on Angina Pectoris caused by atherosclerosis. China Traditional and Western Medicine ER Magazine 1999 Vol. 2 (6).

Lu, G.H., et al. Comparative study of anti-hypertensive effect of Gypenosides, Ginseng and Indapamide in patients with essential hypertension. Guizhou Medical Journal. 1996; 20:1.

Tan, H., et al. Antithrombotic effect of Gynostemma pentaphyllum. Integrated Medicine Journal of China. Chinese. 1993 May; 13(5): 278-280, 261.

Wu, Jiling, et al. Effects of gypenosides on platelet aggregation and camp levels in rabbits. Pharmacology and Toxicology Journal of China. 1990; 4(1): 54-57.

Chen, L.F., et al. Comparison between the effects of gypenosides and gypenosides on cardiac function and hemodynamics in dogs. Pharmacology and Toxicology Journal of China. 1990; 4(1): 17-20.

Zhou, S.R.A Preliminary study on the effects of Gynostemma pentaphyllum on endurance, spontaneous motor activity and superoxide dismutase in mice. Asia Pacific Journal of Pharmacology 1990; 5(4): 321-322.

Arichi, Shigeru, et al. Saponins of Gynostemma pentaphyllum as tonics. Kakai Tokkyo Koho. Jpn. 1985. 60(105): 626.

Tanner MA, et al. The direct release of nitric oxide by gypenosides derived from her Gynostemma pentaphyllum. Nitric Oxide 1999 3(5): 359-65.

Index